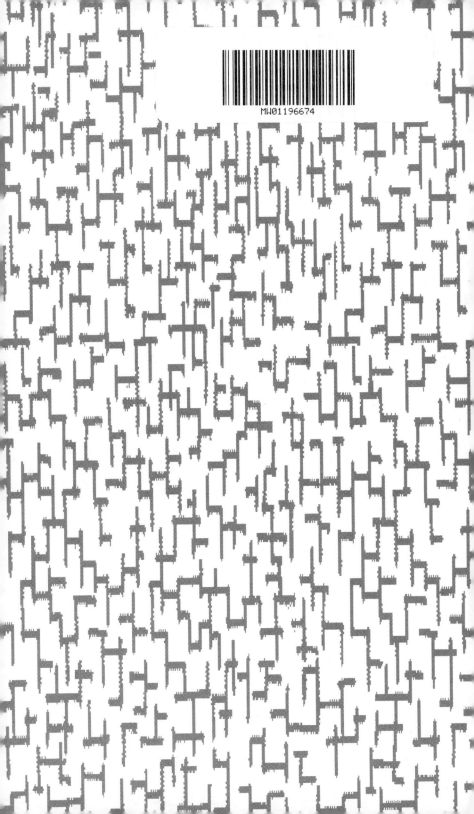

MW01196674

CREATING YOUR PERSONAL
VISION

A MIND-BODY GUIDE
FOR BETTER EYESIGHT

by DR. SAMUEL A. BERNE

COLOR STONE PRESS

SANTA FE, NEW MEXICO

DISCLAIMER

This book is not intended to diagnose, treat, or prescribe. The information contained herein is in no way to be considered a substitute for your own intuition or consultation with a duly licensed health-care professional.

FIRST EDITION

Manufactured in the United States of America
Cover and Text Design by R. Suzanne Vilmain

Library of Congress Catalogue Card Number: 94-72147

ISBN 0-96415599-3-7

Color Stone Press
1300 Luisa St., Suite 4
Santa Fe, New Mexico 87505
505-820-2527

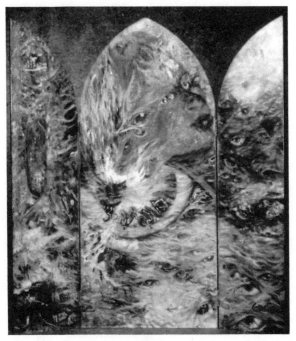

Artist—Georgeanne Jud

*"The first gift beyond that of light was vision,
the inner life of the imagination."* [1]
—**Rowena Pattee Kryder**

CONTENTS

LIST OF ILLUSTRATIONS

ACKNOWLEDGEMENTS

There have been many people who have influenced and helped me with the writing of this book. I'd like to express my gratitude to the teachers who have given me the inspiration to express myself: Drs. A.M. Skeffington, Harry Riley Spitler, Elliot Forrest, Albert Shankman, Ellis Edelman, Richard Apell, Robert Krasken, John Streff, Robert Sanet, Jacob Liberman, Robert-Michael Kaplan, Marc Grossman, Yvonne Kaye, Gerald J. Jud, Hazel Parcells, and Mr. George Bloom.

Thanks to Silver Wave Records, PO Box 7943, Boulder, CO 80306, (303)443-5617 for permission to reprint from the sound recording *Migration* by Peter Kater and R. Carlos Nakai.

Thanks to Element Inc., 42 Broadway, Rockport, MA 01966 and Element Books Ltd, Shaftesbury, Dorset, England for permission to reprint "The Mother's Breath" from *Here to Heal* by Reshad Feild.

Thanks to Sandy Murillo, Wini Bauer, Wendy Ogden, Dr. Gerald J. Jud, Dr. Hazel Parcells, Amadea Morningstar, and Patrick McNamara for permission to reprint interviews and case histories.

Thanks to Bear & Co., Box 2860, Santa Fe, NM 87504 for permission to reprint the quote from *Emerald River of Compassion* by Rowena Pattee Kryder © 1994.

I'd like to thank my brothers, my parents, and all my friends who supported me along the way. I especially thank my editor, Sonya Moore for her expertise, my office manager, Paldrom and our office staff for their commitment to excellence, Charly and Nika for their love and devotion, and my patients who are really *my* teachers. They are a big part of the fabric of this book.

PREFACE

Aldous Huxley in *The Art of Seeing* says, "The doctor treats, nature heals."[2] The conventional medical approach treats symptoms, which only serves to make the causes of illness and malfunction that much more deeply rooted. THE MEDICINE WE NEED IS INSIDE OURSELVES.

In the early 1900s, Dr. W.H. Bates, a New York ophthalmologist, discovered a method to re-educate vision and thus reduce the need to wear glasses. Dr. Bates found that two major causes of vision imbalances were mental tension and poor vision habits.

In 1942, Huxley, expanding on the Bates method of palming, swinging, sunning, and breathing, wrote *The Art of Seeing*, which beautifully described the dynamic process of vision. Huxley observed that seeing was like any other skill—walking, running, talking, playing golf, singing. He postulated that when a serious physical/mental shock occurred to a person, there was often a breakdown in the natural fundamental skill of vision. This breakdown led to inefficient visual habits. By practice, people could regain their vision in a natural way. One of the methods of re-

7

education involved learning to see in a *relaxed* manner, free from strain and mental tension.

Vision improvement also was deeply influenced by some pioneering people in the field of Behavioral Optometry and Vision Therapy.

In the 1920s, A.M. Skeffington, an optometrist, began challenging the current model of vision by asking how the total behavior of a person could be taken into account when prescribing lenses. "Skeff and Associates" continually examined optometric protocol and creatively worked with vision as a global and dynamic system. In 1928, Dr. Skeffington became the Educational Director for the Optometric Extension Program (OEP), which developed information on Behavioral Optometry. Today OEP is a vibrant organization spreading the philosophy and techniques of vision therapy throughout the U.S. and around the world. Dr. Skeffington assembled many distinguished players on his team to explore and experiment with the development of a behavioral vision model:

❖ Professor Samuel Renshaw of Ohio State produced a vision therapy program to help pilots to recognize landmarks and see more quickly when flying missions during WWII.

❖ Professor N. Kaphart, an industrial psychologist, studied the vision of "brain injured" children.

❖ Dr. Darell Boyd Harmon developed theories on the relationship of vision, posture, learning, and human performance.

❖ In the 1940s, Dr. E.B. Alexander, Dr. Frederick Brock, Dr. G.N. Getman, and Dr. Lawrence McDonald experimented with and synthesized vision therapy methods that went beyond straightening crossed eyes. These pioneers built their work partly on the theory of Swiss psychologist Jean Piaget that all children's intellectual development occurred in the same sequential order within distinct stages. Thus a child's cognitive ability could be used as a benchmark to enhance visual abilities related to learning.

In the late 1940s and early 1950s, Dr. Skeffington and Dr. Getman worked with Arnold Gesell at the Yale Clinic of Child Development. It was here that the philosophy of developmental vision care was created. It became apparent from this research that as children began to use their vision more effortlessly, learning, sports, and their relationships became greatly enhanced. One magnificent discovery was that many children who were non-achievers had undetected visual imbalances.

In the mid to late 1950s and 1960s, through the work at the Gesell Institute, Dr. Richard Apell and Dr. John Streff developed programs combining vision, speech and language, psychology, nutrition, and other multi-disciplinary systems to help children reach peak performance. A postgraduate fellowship program was started at the Gesell Institute for practitioners to learn the concepts of Optometric Vision Therapy.

In the 1970s and '80s, Elliot Forrest and Albert Shankman developed the psycho-behavioral model of vision and the Vision Enhancement philosophy.

The ideas and concepts of this book draw not only from this rich lineage but also from the disciplines of biofeedback, nutrition, light and color therapy, homeopathy, naturopathy, Ayurveda, Feldenkrais, Shiatsu, and yoga. When we learn to see effortlessly, there comes a deeper sense of balance and a higher state of wellness. This book is to help you to become an active participant in your health and well-being.

INTRODUCTION

"We must embrace the absurd and go beyond everything we have ever known."[3]
—Janie Gustafson

I turn the key, open the door, turn on the light, and am ready to start another day at the office. I am excited, as I always am, because today I'm going to be helping people see themselves and their world with a new level of clarity and awareness.

Most people are a little scared to be giving up an old habit—their fixed perception. The exciting part is what they have in store for themselves. I remember my own beginning.

❖ ❖ ❖ ❖ ❖ ❖ ❖

I was born in 1957 to a middle class family in Pittsburgh, Pennsylvania. Early in my first few years, both of my parents realized my natural ability to play sports. By 4 years of age, I was already swinging a baseball bat and hitting a golf ball. School was another matter. I really enjoyed the creative work we did in school, but on standardized tests I never did very well. Instead, I preferred to be outside doing physical activities—running and riding my bicycle, being and playing in nature. My parents and teachers thought I didn't like to read and do schoolwork because I was lazy, and that made me a problem learner. When I was forced to read, I was very slow and always had to re-read everything. I could read letters and words, but I tended to lose my place and skip words. That slowed me down. I had poor concentration and became easily frustrated because I couldn't keep up with my classmates. I knew something was wrong with me because I just couldn't read like everyone else. My parents and teachers were as frustrated as I was because my potential and performance never seemed to match. After a while I began to give up because I just couldn't meet everyone's expectations. My escape was to play outside.

When I was 8 my mother took me to the eye doctor. He tested my eyes and said I needed glasses to see far away. I remember sitting in this dark room and feeling very afraid of the man who was examining me. I saw him as another grownup who was going to tell me I was doing something wrong.

He asked me to read some small letters very far away and I couldn't. As so many times before, I felt that I had failed another test. He prescribed some glasses for me and told me that later I would need a stronger prescription. He also told me I would have to wear glasses for the rest of my life. "Great," I thought, "another thing to worry about." Once again my confidence was shaken.

When I put the glasses on, they made my eyes feel tight. Although they helped me see a little clearer, the glasses made my eyes strain to see. It felt like I needed to tense my eyes in order to use them. My parents and teachers said these glasses were the answer to all my learning problems, but in fact I knew deep down that they didn't help me. In fact, the more I looked through these glasses, the worse my eyes felt. They were always tired and hurt a lot after I read with the glasses on.

At about this time, my parents' relationship began to fall apart. The chaos and turmoil made me anxious and afraid. One way to cope with these feelings was to create a boundary to separate me from the world. I hid behind my glasses, becoming very introspective and withdrawn from the external world. It was interesting that as I made the glasses my boundary, the prescription became stronger.

When I was 13, my parents divorced. I know now that I dealt with the confusion by blurring out both my seeing and my feeling. My glasses gave me the sense that I was able to control my chaotic world because seeing clearly with my glasses gave me a sense that my world was exact, neat and tidy, and perfect. Seeing the details meant I knew it all, and I would be rewarded for being so smart. Being acknowledged for getting it all correct made me feel better. As I reflect today on that period of my life, what was really happening was that each time I looked for the detail and pursued "getting it right" the pressure and expectations increased. To compensate I tried harder and tightened my eyes, my mind, and my body. The truth was my glasses gave me the opportunity not to have to see or feel what was really happening to me. They only created an artificial sense of clarity.

My prescription was increased four times in my adolescence. By the time I was 20, I was addicted to my glasses and the behaviors that went with them. I was wearing a nearsighted prescription all the time. My personality was introverted and withdrawn. I was tight and liked to see in one way. I didn't like to give up my point of view.

I entered optometry school in 1980. During my fourth year of school, I had the opportunity to venture away from the classical medical model of the eye. I went to California to spend three months with Dr. Robert Sanet, a Behavioral Optometrist. Dr. Sanet's approach to vision care was through vision therapy, a process I knew very little about. In his office, I saw adults and children coming to practice many different activities that actually improved their vision. Changes ranging from improved school performance in children to improved sports performance for Olympic athletes showed me how potent vision therapy could be.

After my experience with Dr. Sanet, I began experimenting with my own vision prescription, doing vision therapy. As I wore a less powerful and more balanced prescription, I felt relaxation in my eyes and body. My peripheral (side) vision—the intuitive or feeling part of my seeing—began to expand. It is the peripheral vision that gives information on where we have been, where we are now, and where we are going—in other words, orientation in the world. For me, when visual acuity was the only part of my vision that I was aware of, my focus was very one-pointed. The blocked areas of my vision, those I was denying, were precisely where I needed to look.

Most of us, at one time or another, have been prevented from being who we are. Perhaps our feelings have been shut off: "Big boys don't cry," or "Don't get angry, it isn't ladylike." I have observed relationships where people invalidate each other, fearing the other's expression of deepest feelings. For instance, if I express my pain or sadness, it will remind you of your own pain and sadness, which you don't want to acknowledge. If I invalidate you as a way to control you, I don't have to feel. Invalidation only creates separation between people. When we validate another's experience we are giving one of the most powerful healing gifts. Validating is like saying, "Yes, I've felt what you are feeling, so you are not alone."

The glasses we wear represent our attitudes, belief systems, and visual habits, and may not be a true measure of our spiritual seeing. So it becomes critical that as we change our inner vision, we also change the vision we bring into our world.

The great spiritual teachers talk about the path to enlightenment or the path to wholeness. I believe that all of us are already whole and enlightened. We sometimes forget this truth. Conditioning from parents, schools, and culture prevents us from returning to the self. As we improve and expand our vision, we become aware of the conditioning while *simultaneously* seeing our true essence.

Part of being able to see who we really are is matching the inner *vision* with the outer *seeing*.

In my own profession of optometry, I have combined the mathematical and scientific concepts of vision and eyesight with a broader, more holistic approach, exploring how vision impacts total health and well-being.

By using this book, you can experience:

- increased self-confidence
- improved school performance
- longer attention span
- improved skill in following directions
- reading for pleasure
- improved sports performance
- deeper and more intimate relationships
- meeting your potential
- less stress
- improved eye and body comfort
- better sleep
- more emotional stability
- more open-mindedness
- better communication
- inner peace
- reduced dependency on glasses and contacts
- natural visual acuity

No matter what resistance you feel, I encourage you to open your vision to as many levels as possible. Even if you don't wear glasses, you can make your vision multi-dimensional. The way you see is unique and personal to you! Begin to love your vision and yourself.

I am including a "road map" by Peter Kater and R. Carlos Nakai from a sound recording called *Migration*, which you might like to use to help guide you on this journey:

1. Wandering—gathering one's tools.
2. Initiation—preparing oneself.
3. Honoring—recognizing the "sacred" in one's life.
4. Stating Intention—realizing one's purpose.
5. Surrender—letting go of control, allowing vulnerability, leaving what is known.
6. Embracing the Darkness—walking into the unknown, being in the world.
7. Lighting the Flame—conscious connection with spirit.
8. Transformation—climbing the mystic spiral to a vision of oneness, the vision that alters all perceptions.
9. Quietude—listening, observing, being still.
10. Becoming Human—empathy, being in truly responsible relationship.
11. Walking the Path—integrating life experience, teaching by being human.
12. Service—transcendence of the illusion of separateness; joy, humility.[4]

April 7, 1994

Dear Dr. Berne,

Thank you for working with me on improving my vision this past year. When I first came to your office, I was wearing glasses corrected for an astigmatism and with vision of 20/200. The work we did together and the exercises you gave me to do at home made me more aware how stress affects my vision and how I used my glasses as a crutch. I also learned how to see just as well without my glasses.

Last week, I took my eye exam for my driver's license and passed with no eye restrictions for driving! I was elated. Thanks for all of your help. Your work is truly outstanding.

Sincerely,

Patrick McNamara

REFERENCE WORDS
CHAPTER ONE

VISION: the act of sensing with the eyes, the mind, and the body. It is a learned skill that develops in a sequence of predictable stages. Sight (visual acuity, i.e. 20/20) is *one* aspect of vision.

MACULA: central part of the retina where detail and clarity of sight and color awareness occur.

DIOPTER: unit of measure that describes the power of a lens or optical system (such as the eye).

ACUITY: sharpness, distinctness, clearness that is dependent on retinal focus.

MIRRORING: reporting back in an objective manner what another person has said or done.

INTUITION: the art of knowing without rational process.

CREATING YOUR PERSONAL VISION

A NEW DIRECTION OF VISION CARE

*"We do a lot of looking: we look through
lenses, telescopes, television tubes. . . .
Our looking is perfected every day—
but we see less and less."*[5]
—**Frederick Franck**

Fifty-eight-year-old Lisa came into the office recently with a personal revelation: "I finally understand how changing my awareness has helped me start using the *vision* I was ignoring all these years. I am beginning to give everything equal attention instead of just focusing on the retinal degeneration that has caused me so much anguish. I feel integrated, connected, and whole for the first time."

Lisa and I had been working together for about two months. Objectively, she had expanded her visual field by 25 percent. Her focusing skills and eye teaming abilities had improved to the level where she could read again.

Through the work we had done together, Lisa realized she still had some *macula* intact in each eye. (Physically the macula is the part of the retina where we see detail. It has to do with intention and being able to sustain focus.) When Lisa first came to see me with her macular degeneration diagnosis, she was afraid she would lose her freedom because she wouldn't be able to see to drive. She was losing her purpose in life. By regaining some vision and learning to use what she had remaining to the best of her ability, Lisa rekindled her life's energy.

Barbara, a 37-year-old massage therapist described her vision in this way: "I understand that my nearsightedness caused me to separate myself from others. I was afraid to interact with people because they would see who I was and wouldn't like me. I thought if I just focused on details, I could avoid the pain of not feeling loved. Improving my vision has been the most empowering aspect in my life. As I reduce my prescription I am able to see more of the truth in myself and others."

When Barbara first came to see me she was wearing -10.00 *diopters* in each eye. This means she could see clearly about 3 inches in front of her face. Barbara chose massage therapy as her profession to help release the stress and tension in her own body. She perceives most of the stress she now has is carried in her eyes. Barbara knows if she can learn to change her visual habits much of this tension will be released. She has been working in vision therapy for three months. In that time she has reduced the power of her prescription by 30 percent.

Initially, I asked Barbara (as I ask everyone who wants to work with me) why she wanted to improve her eyesight and vision. She said, "I know I'm seeing through some very strong filters that have frozen my vision and limited my awareness. No matter how much healing I do on myself, I am still stuck in my perceptions. I'm ready to change the way I see." I have heard comments like these many times from patients, and I am convinced that healing, on whatever level, is a vibrant, holistic, and complex process.

In a clinical situation, I have found there are five vital components necessary for healing to occur. First, the patient needs to be seen and heard. This means validating persons for *who they are*. A space is created for them to feel safe. Second, it is important for the healer to present possibilities to the patient for continued enhancement and growth, exuding encouragement and support. Third, both healer and patient *must* enter into a partnership for healing. One of my early teachers told me that vision therapy is about the therapist setting up the conditions for a person to work on vision improvement. There needs to be clear communication: *the therapist does not heal the patient*. On the contrary, patients take the responsibility for causing their own healing. As Deepak Chopra says: "All of us have the medicine inside ourselves to do our own healing."[6]

The next essential component in the healing process is that the healer go through his or her own transformation. Experiencing one's own healing brings a deep belief that anyone can improve and heal themselves. When the healer deeply and authentically believes the healing process, the patient will be more inclined to embark on the same process. Going through vision therapy as a patient has given me insights, wisdom, and compassion for those I work with today.

When I started my practice of optometry in 1984, I was wearing my sixth pair of glasses in 20 years. Although I had been educated quite extensively in the medical model of vision and the science of optometry, I questioned this model as being the only way to improve a person's vision. I was especially interested in how the lenses I was taught to prescribe affected a person on many levels: physiologically, psychologically, emotionally, and spiritually.

The science of optometry trains optometrists to correct a person's blurry vision optically by putting a lens in front of the eye to focus the light on the retina. When the light focuses exactly on the retina, a person should have 20/20 *acuity*, which means being able to read a 1/3" letter at 20 feet. Optics says that in nearsightedness (myopia), the light entering the eye focuses in front of the retina and a *minus* lens is needed to refocus on the retina. In farsightedness (hyperopia), the light focuses behind the retina and a *plus* lens is needed to refocus on the retina. In astigmatism part of the light focuses in front and part behind the retina so a combination lens is needed to refocus the light. *(For a more complete explanation, see pages 62-66.)*

Although mathematically this philosophy works well, I felt all I was doing for people was artificially compensating for blur. Since I then wore a pair of glasses that corrected for blur, I began to experiment with my own vision. I reduced my prescription by 20 percent, began doing vision exercises through this reduced prescription, and began improving my nutrition and practicing yoga and meditation. I started to experience awareness changes similar to those my patients were reporting in their own vision improvement programs—for example, more mental and emotional flexibility. I didn't stay stuck on one perspective for as long as I used to. I experienced more feelings. My creativity improved. I began to listen more and follow my intuition (inner feelings). I felt less stressed and had more energy to live my life. As a vision therapist, I found the deeper I could go with my *own* vision improvement, the deeper I could take my patients with *their* own vision improvement.

I have experienced a healing power when men get together and are able to share their feelings with each other. I thought this healing energy could be used in the doctor-patient relationship. Instead of the doctor telling the patient, "This is what is wrong with you," perhaps the doctor could act as a mirror for patients to help guide them where they need to heal. *Mirroring* means simply that I report back to you what you have said or done in an objective manner for you to see yourself. Lynn Andrews, who has studied with Native American medicine women says, "mirroring the life force of our patients helps them see themselves."[7]

Self-awareness in the patient is a powerful curative factor. Many patients I have worked with have developed their *inner* vision by spiritual practices like meditation, yoga, or the martial arts, but there often is a lag in the *outer* seeing. On this path, it is important to change our outer seeing to match our inner vision or old habits and conditioning come back.

The last condition for healing involves loving. Dr. Gerald J. Jud, a leader in the human potential movement and founder of Shalom Mountain Retreat and Study Center speaks of loving as an art that involves skills that can be learned. These skills are: seeing, listening and hearing, expressing good will, recognizing each person's right to think and feel as they do, and being fully present to another human.[8]

Self-love must precede loving others. There must be compassion toward one's own needs and vulnerability. Judgment and advice giving only create separation and are not part of love. Love gives an open space for persons to explore their true essence, recognizing their own uniqueness. When love is present, the magic of healing can occur because an open space of safety is created for each person's exploration and discovery journey.

Recently, Kerry came in for an initial consultation. She described the process of her glasses being made thicker and thicker as she was growing up. She was presently wearing -14.00 diopters for both eyes. She had become very angry at her eye doctors for she felt that the constant increase of her prescription was only making her eyes more dependent on the glasses.

She began crying, then remembered asking one eye doctor if he could reduce her prescription. He said "No," that because of her vision problems there was no alternative except to increase the strength of the glasses, thus invalidating her questions and concerns.

I related the five components for healing to Kerry's past experience with her vision care. The doctors she had been to had not experienced improvement in their own vision. They were caught in the habit of seeing only one approach. When Kerry had suggested she wanted to participate in healing her vision, the doctors could only offer the traditional method.

Kerry felt she just couldn't go any further in the relationship with those doctors. The love space was not present so her healing couldn't occur.

The traditional method is treatment with a symptom approach, but when only symptoms are treated, the imbalance is driven further into the person. Using the symptom approach is trying to perform a "quick fix" or use a "magic bullet"—a conventional cover-up that masks the true problem. Using vision therapy, Kerry has the option to change her vision and her prescription, which in three months has improved 25 percent. Kerry is committed to continue expanding and improving her vision and totally reducing the dependency on her glasses.

Although patients come into the office with the intention of reducing such dependency, the essence of creating personal vision is learning to see in an effortless, natural way. However, before a person can experience effortless vision, he or she needs to understand present visual habits. Most people are unaware of how they use their vision; and glasses only support this lack of awareness. When we begin to take our glasses off or wear a reduced prescription, we can observe how our blur changes based on stress, emotions, thoughts, and nutrition. Therefore, we can use our vision as a wonderful biofeedback device that gives us a road map on where we need to do our healing. The visual exercises and light therapy act as a mirror, which shows us the visual habits we've developed to use in our interactions with the world.

In continuing my vision improvement, I realized that vision isn't just in the eyes. The practice of yoga and the development of more body awareness helped me see with every cell in my body—whole body seeing. I noticed that my visual field became constricted when I was operating most rationally, whereas if I became more body-centered, my visual field expanded greatly. The less I worried about getting it right, the more I went into the process and beyond the process.

When I took my glasses off I initially felt very anxious and afraid. I realized that these were the same feelings I'd had when I got my first pair of glasses. Staying with these feelings, I began to bring up other memories and emotions.

Glasses sharpened the way of seeing through the eyes of my ego. Being able to follow my inner knowing was conflicting and confusing for me. "Besides," my ego asked, "why do I have to change anything and follow some unexplainable inner feeling? I see clearly—I see everything clearly, therefore I know it all and I am perfect already." Yet, all that time I was *really insecure and unsure* about what I saw, so I began the habit of straining, looking harder to make myself feel more secure. Seeing an external object clearly through my glasses was a way to trust myself. The glasses I wore kept me focused externally, out of my body. That way I could avoid my feelings.

I became aware that my nearsightedness was supported by my fear of seeing parts of myself. I was hiding a part of myself for fear of not being accepted and loved. I felt nobody was able to understand me or support what I wanted to do. Sometimes when I observed others around me, I internalized their behaviors and expectations through my eyes, then projected these behaviors and expectations out into the world. Nearsightedness has to do with freezing these experiences and not being able to dissolve them easily.

The glasses I saw through kept my vision narrow and tight. Improving my vision gave me the opportunity to release these energies, to gain the flexibility to see from another perspective. Only when I began to take my glasses off did trust come more from inside, from my inner vision. When I looked with blurred vision, initially I felt frustration, fear, uncertainty, out of control. I began to see just how *dependent* I had become on my glasses. As I began to relax into the blur instead of fighting it, my side-vision began to open up, and I realized taking the glasses off afforded me another perspective. This insight was very empowering to me.

Today I have learned that the less effort I use to see, the more aware I am. The harder I try, the more stress I feel, and the less I see. Often, what I'm missing is precisely where I need to put my attention.

Some of the characteristics of acuity-oriented, sharp, narrow, focused attitudes and behaviors are:

❖ Lack of flexibility and adaptability, and difficulty in flowing with the energy of life.

❖ Answer-oriented, grade-oriented, product-oriented approach with little thought to being present to the process.

❖ Fear-based need to control the external world.

❖ Focusing externally, and losing awareness of internal focus.

❖ Being overly critical and judgmental about oneself and others.

The first part of "creating your personal vision" is to become aware of visual conditioning and habits. The second part is to reconnect and integrate vision with the rest of awareness, so that seeing becomes a total full-body process, involving movement and action. This connection can have a profound effect on every aspect of our lives.

As I continue the journey of improving my vision, I see more softly and behave more gently. I continue to learn how many psychological and emotional components there are to how we create our personal vision.

After I graduated from optometry school and completed my experience with Dr. Sanet in California, I knew that I wanted to work with people to help them improve their vision. I decided to open an office in the western suburbs of Philadelphia, found some great office space in a restored historic building, and arranged to get financing from the bank. However, right before the deal was to close the financing fell through and I lost that opportunity.

Feeling very discouraged, I was driving around the area when I saw a sign that read "Dr. E.S. Edelman, Visual Perceptual Therapy." A few months before I had written to this man asking if I could come and visit his office sometime. Something inside me said, "Why not now?"

Dr. Edelman was not busy so I introduced myself. I told him about my experience working in Dr. Sanet's vision therapy office in San Diego, and that I wanted to specialize in this area of optometry. He began describing the model of vision that he had developed over his thirty years of practice. Although some of the concepts were new to me, I was fascinated by what Dr. Edelman was saying. By the end of the meeting, I asked to come into his office, pay rent, and start my own practice, and he was agreeable to this suggestion.

As I reflect today on what happened, my failure to get a bank loan to open my office was just a guidepost that led to the opportunity with Dr. Edelman. The whole series of events felt effortless. It seems that the part of me that is my inner knowing actually led me there.

What I have learned is that this inner feeling called the *intuition* comes when we are not forcing or straining. When we strain to make something happen, we actually block our intuition, our higher intelligence, so to speak. Many times we may get an intuitive impulse, but fear and worry (our rational thinking at work) get in the way and we don't follow that impulse. It comes down to trusting our intuition, trusting what we see and feel.

In my early adult years, I confused intuition with my mind and emotions. The distinction comes from learning about the different parts of ourselves. Spiritual practices such as yoga, T'ai Chi, and meditation can help us become aware of these different parts. As we go deeper in our self-exploration, it becomes easier for us to distinguish between thoughts and emotions (based on conditioning) and intuition (the higher intellegence part of us).

As an experiment, for the next week, whenever you are feeling confused or indecisive about what to do, ask yourself in a yes/no fashion whether you should do it or not. Make it simple, like: Should I go for a run today? Should I call this person? As you ask the question, listen for the first answer. Follow that answer and notice how you feel as you follow through. Notice how you feel when you don't follow through. Begin to trust your first impulse and notice the clarity and power you experience.

REFERENCE WORDS
CHAPTER TWO

GIFTED CHILDREN: commonly labeled as "handi-capped" or "challenged", these children with multiple handicaps or visual impairment are truly gifted and frequently very spiritually evolved.

CORTICAL BLINDNESS: the brain is unable to inter-pret the messages sent by the eyes.

RETINOSCOPY: procedure that measures the bending of light into one's eyes.

AGE-RELATED MACULAR DEGENERATION (ARMD): a vision loss in the central part of the retina.

PERIPHERAL VISION: vision to the sides of the head, assisting in one's balance and movement in space.

SUPPRESSION: an adaptation in which all or part of the visual input of one eye is prevented from contribut-ing to binocular (two-eyed) vision.

TRUSTING OUR VISION

*"It is only with the heart that one can see rightly;
what is essential is invisible to the eye."*[9]
—Antoine de Saint-Exupery

The wearing of glasses is based on habits and conditioning. I used my own glasses as a boundary, a protection from my surroundings. I could hide my insecurity behind them.

Ed, one of my patients, gave me some insights into why he developed his nearsightedness (-11.00 diopters).

"I grew up in a family that was very poor. My father was never home because he was always at work. I had four brothers and two sisters, so my mother was too busy to be there for me. I used to spend most of the time in my head, thinking. My thoughts and ideas were my friends. In vision therapy I have realized how addicted I am to being mental. This behavior has been a way for me to escape the pain and

35

loneliness I must have felt growing up. I've certainly missed out on many experiences in my life."

There is a correlation between the mental chatter, which could be worry or unfocused thinking, and the glasses we wear. In Ed's case, for example, his glasses acted as a filter that blocked his life experience because it was painful. He altered his perception by using thinking as a way to distract him from what was really happening in front of his eyes. As we remain distracted by the mental chatter, our total awareness—including intuition—decreases. Guidance then comes from an external stimulus or from our thoughts or emotions instead of from our higher intelligence.

In my first year of practice, my intuition was tested as a whole new area of using vision therapy opened for me. I began to attract patients with traumatic brain injury and closed head trauma. These people had tremendous visual problems. I could not find any research on using vision therapy as a form of treatment, but our results were so favorable that I performed my own research. I published the information to let other practitioners know there were other options available.

One such case involved a 22-year-old woman named Lois. Six weeks previously she had been in an auto accident and hit her head on the dashboard. When Lois came for her first visit, she was complaining of double vision, poor balance, and difficulty with concentration and memory. She had been told that the only options available were to have surgery to correct the double vision or to wear an eye patch. What Lois really wanted was to be able to read again and to go back to her job.

I explained that her head injury had caused a functional change in her vision. By going through the process of vision therapy, Lois could relearn how to use her brain and body. We worked together with vision therapy, improving her awareness and the function of her visual skills. Techniques using the colored flashlight, the Marsdan ball, the Brock String, and parquetry designs (*see chapters 5 and 6*), were designed as visual problem-solving to give her awareness of vision, concentration, movement, and memory.

After we had worked for three months, Lois's occupational therapist called to say she was amazed with the behavioral and emotional changes in Lois. Thus, for me, began the marriage between occupational therapy and vision therapy.

This relationship is such a natural combination. In people with traumatic brain injury, stroke, and multi-handicaps, the rehabilitation process can be painfully slow. What seems to work in therapy is for the healer to "tune into" the patient, starting where that person is going to be receptive. Many therapists and doctors want to impose their own method or approach on a patient. Schools tend to do this as well—teaching only in one way. If the person doesn't fit into that mode, he or she won't be helped within that system.

A method I like to use involves engaging in an activity and seeing how the patient responds. Then the next activity is based on that response. I watch the eyes, the body, and the posture as I am working. I use my own past experience and my intuition and I mirror back—reflect—the response so the patient develops better self-awareness.

An example of this occurred recently with Carol. As she was reading the arrow chart (*see pages 110-112*), I noticed her hand motions were very small. So I had her march out the directions with her whole body to help her become aware of how habitually restricted her movement is. Once she realized this pattern, the exercise went from being boring to being fun. In rehabilitation especially, care needs to be taken to start where the person is and to be open and creative, changing the method to fit the person.

GIFTED CHILDREN

An example involves my work with several *gifted children*. Labels are placed on these children: they have minimal brain dysfunction or attention deficit disorder or cortical blindness. Most of society doesn't know how to handle these cases. Parents are often devastated to hear these labels. They believe there is no hope for healing with such a diagnosis, when, in reality, a label only means that the child does not fit into the doctor's or school's belief system.

Danny, a 4-year-old, severely brain injured child was brought in by his parents with a diagnosis of *cortical blindness*. This term really intrigues me. What does it mean? The person has no light perception? The brain cells are blind? Is there any usable vision? I believe this is a catch-all term used by professionals because they can't measure the amount of vision available by using traditional methods (like the visual acuity chart). Probably we all often use labels as a way to make ourselves feel better. I believe placing labels on people identifies them for life. Categorizing someone's potential keeps a lid on their growth.

My *retinoscopy* of Danny revealed a moderate amount of nearsightedness (- 4.00), some intermittent fixation with both eyes (he could maintain focus on an object intermittently), and 80 percent usable peripheral vision. Danny and his parents felt a sense of validation and healing in finding that he had usable vision. His parents told me I was the first male doctor/healer he had worked with. On Danny's first visit I had his parents take his leg braces off and the two of us jumped together on the trampoline for 15 minutes. Danny's joy at being so freely active was overflowing.

Using the trampoline with Danny gave him the freedom to move his body. The leg braces symbolized restriction; yet his nature was to be in movement. Parents need to be given a choice when the professional prescribes glasses, leg braces, or medication. In this case, jumping on the trampoline gave Danny (and his parents) another perspective on how to be in the world. Working closely with Danny's teachers and occupational therapist has been a wonderful opportunity to watch Danny grow and begin to explore his world.

I believe another aspect to working with these gifted children is connecting with the spirit. Generally, they are very spiritually evolved, highly intuitive, creative beings and they need to be recognized for these characteristics.

This recognition is an important opening with them. Combining recognition with the ability to work, gearing my technique to their level, is a key for healing. Acceptance, openness, and partnership are important ingredients for success.

ARMD

The elderly who become partially-sighted are another segment of the population who need more attention. One of the most common diseases facing these people is *age-related macular degeneration (ARMD)*.

The retina lines the inner eyeball and is a light-sensitive membrane. When light enters the eye and reaches the retina, chemical impulses are created, which go to the brain and allow us to see. In the anatomy of the eye, there are two parts of the retina—the macula and the peripheral retina. The peripheral part gives us side vision. It is located slightly to the outside of the center of the retina. The most inner portion of the macula, the fovea centralis, contains densely packed cells called the cones. These cells, aside from giving us detailed vision, also are responsible for our color vision. It is interesting that no direct blood vessels run through the macula; it gets nourishment from other retinal blood vessels.

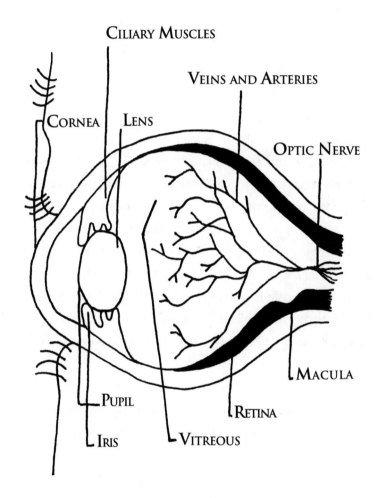

CILIARY MUSCLES

VEINS AND ARTERIES

CORNEA LENS

OPTIC NERVE

MACULA

PUPIL

RETINA

IRIS

VITREOUS

ANATOMY OF THE EYE

Illustration by Michelle Goodman

In macular degeneration, there is improper circulation occurring through the macula. It can either become dried out or have too much fluid around it. Pigment changes can also affect the function of the macula. Macular degeneration can be quite devastating because, with a loss of visual acuity, many older people will not be able to drive anymore. This loss is a real symbol of losing independence. Reading also becomes more difficult and any nearpoint detail work is not possible.

The common stance is that nothing can really help; but I have found that much can be done. The key with macular degeneration is to show people how much vision they have remaining (usually the peripheral vision) and teach them to put this vision to the best possible use. It may mean moving the head and/or body in order to see. It may mean using a low-vision aid such as a telescope to see road signs or a magnifying glass to see small print. It may mean becoming more flexible in using vision. These people must be willing to try new ways to best utilize the vision they have.

The *peripheral vision* is one of the most important functions of the vision system. Peripheral vision is the foundation for understanding time, size, and spatial relationships. It helps a person integrate movement and balance. When the peripheral vision is not being used, a person can be "accident prone," lose the place when reading, have poor copying ability, and generally be unsure about moving through the world. Vision therapy is an excellent way to help a person develop more peripheral vision.

People with ARMD see the world as a blur, one which cannot be corrected with lenses. This blurriness can be unnerving because it is a different way of seeing. Many times fear sets in and they will tense and tighten, contract and close down. They feel their vision/their eyes are something outside themselves, out of their control. It almost becomes a paralysis. When we focus more on the fear, on what is wrong, these thoughts become habitual.

Stress plays a role in the way a person uses vision. The ARMD patient may need to learn stress reduction and relaxation exercises. Learning that they do have control over their vision and health is a major key for success.

It is interesting that when I begin helping people let go of their thoughts, they don't want to. They have more fear about the emptiness that replaces the fear thoughts, than of the actual fear thoughts themselves. *Where will the mind go next?* is a common fear.

One of my colleagues once said that 95 percent of the thoughts we have today will be the same tomorrow and the next day—and most of them are meaningless. There is a correlation between these thoughts and our vision: when we think, we focus, we narrow in, so our peripheral vision shrinks and our total awareness contracts.

Patients with ARMD can learn to see with the whole body, not just with their eyes. One exercise involves reading an arrow chart in time with a metronome (*see pages 110-112*), an activity taken from work on stress therapy by Dr. Robert Pepper. You move your hands in the direction of the arrows with the beat of the metronome, using the exercise to mirror your own awareness. Part of that awareness involves being able to move your body and your hands *and* concentrate on reading at the same time. When the mind is engaged with mental chatter, you won't be able to do the activity effortlessly. Only when you let go of the chatter and begin to trust yourself by letting the activity happen without controlling or forcing the results, can vision become effortless.

Integrating vision and movement is about having relaxed attention. This relaxed attention supports expanded awareness, which is in fact an expansion of peripheral vision. This is just what a person with ARMD needs to focus on. My experience is that as the periphery improves, acuity will also improve. As mentioned in chapter 1, someone who is focused only on seeing clearly is very answer-oriented. The fear and focus are on getting it right. However, by learning to relax and see with less acuity, many other aspects of vision besides the peripheral will open. This opening supports a more relaxed and effortless way to see.

Whole-body seeing involves seeing from your center, as in the martial art of Aikido where the masters speak of coming from the center or one-point. From a vision standpoint, when your seeing comes from the true one-point, your vision opens up. The one-point is not about seeing with the eyes only, however. The best way to visualize this is with the arrow chart—every part of the body "sees" from the center at the solar plexus. Since vision is awareness and you can experience this awareness through your whole body, when you see in this way your perception becomes totally connected to what you are doing. Your energy is working in alignment and this is when effortlessness happens. This is experiencing yourself in the spaces between your thoughts.

STRABISMUS

One of the most interesting visual conditions is strabismus. Sometimes referred to as cross-eyed (eyes turning in) or wall-eyed (eyes turning out), strabismus is a condition where one eye fixates on an object while the other eye points in a different direction. The eyes don't work together. Many times this lack of integration in the eyes is also reflected in a lack of integration between the hemispheres of the brain and the lack of integration between both sides of the body.

The reasons for strabismus can be many-fold. A difficult birth, a childhood trauma or sickness, even tumors, strokes, or nerve/brain damage can cause a strabismus. There have been some cases of strabismus taking place while the fetus is in utero. There is constant vibrational communication between mother and child that can have a profound effect on the child's perception. If the messages from the mother are mixed or not clear, the child can begin to develop mismatches in perception even before birth. Many eye doctors blame strabismus on weak eye muscles which control eye movements. Behavioral Optometry believes that it is the *brain* that regulates the eye movement by *directing* the eye muscles. In order to treat strabismus one must first realize that it is a symptom of a deeper problem. For example, a child could become cross-eyed as a way to focus inwardly (as a type of compensation). Or, the eyes could focus apart because the child becomes stressed out trying to focus-in (the child is lost in space, not sure where he or she is and where to look). In both cases, the child has a lack of awareness and control of how to coordinate the eyes and body.

Working on a brain level (which vision therapy addresses) is more effective than trying to treat strabismus by altering the length of the muscles through surgery. There are many psychological and emotional factors relating to why a person develops strabismus as an adaptation to seeing the world. There is usually a state of confusion and fear with little or no sense of relationship to their world; in short, people with strabismus don't know where they are in space. Cross-eyed people usually see the world in one fixed way. Wall-eyed people see the world with many points of view. There is difficulty making decisions because they cannot focus-in on one answer.

The underlying key for success in treating strabismus is to reprogram the brain so the eyes, the brain, and the body work together in a more holistic, integrated manner. The first aspect in reprogramming is to help patients become aware of the old messages and habits that caused the strabismus. This may mean having them either vocalize or write down all of their mental chatter. Most of this chatter has been internalized because people weren't permitted to share their feelings as children. A common belief system is: "I don't feel safe enough to share myself, so I'll keep everything inside of me." This blocked energy needs to come out.

When both eyes are not aimed at the same object as in strabismus, the person becomes an expert at *suppression*. Suppression is an adaptation the brain has made to control the eye muscles, so that instead of seeing double, one of the visual inputs has been mentally shut off by the brain. This helps the person avoid the conflicting inputs the eyes are seeing. A person suppressing one of their visual inputs literally can also be shutting off that side of the brain and the body, the emotions and perceptions, and the awareness. Some symptoms of suppression can be: confusion of words (reversals), a conflict in decision making, or an inability to problem-solve. Suppression can cause a rigidity in perceptions or a denial of emotions. A person with strabismus deals with their condition by either grappling with two realities or disregarding one of them. Suppressing part of the outer seeing only reflects that part of the inner vision they must deny. To do this requires an incredible amount of energy. Vision therapy gives a person permission to see and feel in a new and expanded way. Being able to use both eyes together effortlessly helps a person create inner peace.

One technique I have developed to encourage visual coordination is an opportunity to experience awareness with each eye. The procedure is called eye dialogue. The patient sits comfortably with one eye patched. I then ask him or her to speak through the unpatched eye, to speak on perceptions, feelings, or whatever comes; not to think about what to say, but just to speak spontaneously. One question I like to ask each eye is how old the eye feels when it sees. Usually the age that is reported relates to the time when part of the person shut down because of a traumatic event, such as the birth of a sibling. The perceptual filter that the person "sees through" feels very young, even though chronologically the person may be an adult.

I also relate each eye to the Chinese medicine model: the right eye symbolizes the father/masculine energy, the left eye symbolizes the mother/feminine energy. The energy relates not only within the person but also as it is projected outward. Below is a list of some of the characteristics of the masculine and feminine energetic relationship.

MASCULINE	FEMININE
Left brain	Right brain
Action-oriented	Intuitive
Forging ahead	Receptive
Focused	Holistic
Goal-oriented	Nourishing
Firm	Spatial
Assertive	Artistic
Adventuresome	Feeling
Industrious	Creative
Initiating	Sensing

The key to living in a harmonious and creative way is to have a union between the feminine and masculine energies. When our eyes are working together, there is an incredible feeling of being strong and open, full of wisdom, with peace, power, and love flowing through. Ultimately this occurs when our inner vision matches the outer seeing.

Steve, a 38-year-old psychotherapist, came to see me for his lazy right eye, which was diagnosed when he was 5 years old. During our initial testing, Steve could not believe how shut down his right eye was. When I patched his left eye and we did the eye dialogue procedure through his right eye, Steve felt his right eye was seeing like a 3 year old. He remembered his father's energy, which was very violent and chaotic. Steve then had a memory of his father whipping his brother while he watched and an incredible amount of pain and sadness overcame him. He started crying, something his father never allowed. Steve admitted he was very disconnected from his own masculine energy. We worked almost two months on the emotional aspects of Steve's vision. We started using the physical exercises of vision therapy, and Steve's visual acuity in his right eye improved from 20/50 to 20/25. I believe that going to the core issues allowed a clearing for Steve and created a deeper healing for him.

On a physical level of vision, it is important for the patient to experience seeing with both eyes simultaneously even if they aren't aiming at the same place. One exercise I use involves prism glasses that create double vision.

Seeing two objects while using the special prism glasses is a mirroring device that allows a patient to process old suppressed memories and feelings. Working through those feelings, he or she must maintain two targets. It is the suppressed energy that is a major factor in the strabismus. When these feelings come into the patient's awareness, it is very important that he or she experience them. Once these memories and feelings are expressed, it becomes easier to develop binocular vision (the eyes working together and aiming at the same place).

Jean was a 37-year-old artist who suffered from an intermittent divergent strabismus (eyes turn out) and amblyopia (a lazy left eye). Her lazy left eye was diagnosed when she was 4 years old. Jean was wearing a pair of farsighted glasses (+2.50 diopters in the right eye and +3.50 diopters in the left eye). Her best corrected visual acuity in the left eye was 20/80; it was 20/20 in the right eye. Jean was very frustrated with her vision. "I just went back to my eye doctor and she said my eyes have gotten worse, I need a stronger prescription, and I'm going to need to wear glasses for the rest of my life." As an artist Jean relied on her vision. She wanted to participate in healing it.

Jean and I started therapy using the prism glasses as one of the first exercises. As Jean looked through these glasses, she couldn't believe how shut down her left eye was; the right eye did all the work. Some very deep feelings came up about her mother as she continued to look. "I feel anger and sadness because my mother wasn't supporting me as a child." She said she felt deprived, then began to grieve and cry about this loss. As we explored the eye dialogue, Jean found that she "took on" the relationship of her parents when she was a 6 year old: her right eye felt domineering, angry, and rigid; her left eye felt out of control, very scared, and unfocused. Each time Jean experienced her eyes individually, her vision would become clearer.

I began doing the arrow exercise with Jean to help her develop better integration between her eyes, her brain, and her body. At first the exercise felt like school—her only focus was to perform and get it right. Then she did the exercise with just her left eye. I had her continue to move back until the arrows were blurry, then read them. Finally she could read them 14 feet away!

Although she saw with the left eye in a softer way, Jean realized her lazy eye was connected to conditioning and limited belief systems. The left eye shutting down, an inability to access her deep feminine nature, painful relationships with others—it was all beginning to fit. As Jean worked through these memories and feelings, I had her practice teaming her eyes together using a Brock String. Jean was able to look at each bead on the string and maintain the "X"—that is seeing two strings going into the bead she was looking at and two strings leaving that bead. For the first time she felt integrated and connected within herself.

Jean brought me one of her paintings, which was very vibrant, alive, and passionate, exactly how she said she was feeling since starting to use her eyes together. She improved the visual acuity in her left eye from 20/80 to 20/30. I reduced her prescription to +1.25 diopters in each eye. I explained to Jean that her old prescription actually froze the ability to focus and kept her old visual habits in place. The new prescription was supporting her ability to do some of the focusing, and encouraging symmetry between her eyes. The principle is that if we give the body a chance to come into balance, it will. When old memories and emotions are cleared, it becomes easier to stay in balance.

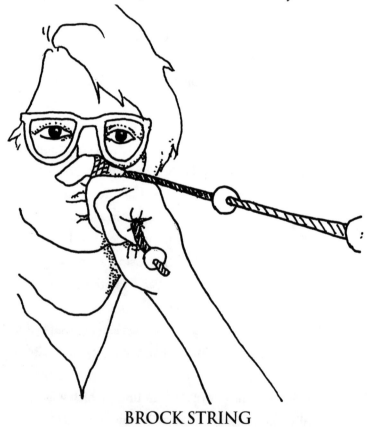

BROCK STRING

Illustration by Michelle Goodman

One option for strabismus is surgery, cutting the muscles so the eyes appear cosmetically straight. There are many drawbacks and disadvantages with this approach. First, the surgery is a symptom-oriented answer to the problem. Cutting the muscles scrambles the signal from the eyes to the brain. As this communication is distorted, the person loses control of the eye muscles. Surgery also inhibits the natural connection between the eyes and brain.

What tends to happen is that the eye will appear straight for a short period of time, but the brain and the body continue to function as though the eye is still turned. The eye tends to revert back to its original condition. Sometimes it even moves in the opposite direction; the brain and body think the eye is in, but the eye wanders out. In essence, a mismatch, a misperception, or a conflict has been created within the person. The brain and the eyes are operating from two different points of view.

In general, people with a strabismus tend to internalize the stress in their vision. The message is, "I cannot trust my vision, I cannot trust what I see. After all, something must be wrong with the way I see, which is why I need surgery. I feel invalidated in the way I see. I am ashamed and embarrassed that my eyes don't look straight." The psychoemotional effects of this kind of surgery can be devastating. The person seems to be very confused about his or her inner awareness. The trauma of the surgery seems to block this inner awareness. Usually feelings of inadequacy, low self-esteem, and shame are present. The person is embarrassed to make eye contact, yet in our culture making eye contact is one of the ways to communicate intimately.

The postsurgical strabismus patient also has trouble with orientation in space. "I don't know where I am in relationship to my world," is a common statement. If the eyes don't straighten in the first surgery, many times the surgeon wants to perform the surgery again. This attempt only creates more confusion between the eyes and the brain.

The surgery covers up the basis of the problem. In order for healing to occur, the person's vision needs to be validated. Postsurgical strabismus patients need to be given lots of love and support. They are usually very fearful and sensitive and need to process their feelings about their surgery. Patients may report double vision or may have certain perceptions about what they see during vision therapy. It is *crucial* that they be told that it is OK to see whatever they see. Everybody needs to create their vision as they wish.

It has been my experience that when I can work on a deeper core level with people, the results are more real and lasting. Performing mechanical exercises alone is not enough. Strabismus is an eye coordination difficulty based on strong visual conditioning. The strabismus is deeply connected to a person's self-image and projection of that self into the world. A large component involves psychoemotional factors. The keys for assisting the process in healing involve being present, loving without judgment, and being a mirror for self-discovery. It is the self-discovery that is empowering for the patient. No fancy psychotherapeutic techniques are needed. *But,* to be effective the vision therapist must do his/her own healing. As one of my strabismus patients said to me, "Vision therapy has helped me put my world together!"

REFERENCE WORDS
CHAPTER THREE

PERCEPTION: an intuition, knowledge or insight gained by perceiving. Perception is the product of perceiving. It is an interpretation of inputs which can be influenced by the accuracy or inaccuracy of inputs (from the eyes), past experiences, personality, memory, and decision-making ability. Perception is a skill we acquire and can be distorted by the mind. These distortions create warps in perception.

DYSLEXIA: lack of coordination and communication between body systems, often causing difficulty in learning to spell and read.

HOW IS YOUR VISION? A SELF-ANALYSIS

*"Albert Schweitzer became indignant when
he noticed I was drawing him with his glasses on:
'Don't please, they make me look so old!'
He was eighty-six..."*[10]
—**Frederick Franck**

To improve vision, it is very important to understand why we see in a certain way. When we have an experience that triggers a *perception*, but the experience is distorted by the mind, then the perception will be distorted as well. An example of this involved a 10-year-old boy named Barry who came in complaining of difficulties in reading. During the evaluation, his eyes were not working together and he experienced double vision. He said he saw double (his perception) every time he tried to read. His experience of reading became one of struggle, pain, and avoidance, and he felt dumb.

In vision therapy, I worked with Barry to help him reduce the double vision, and reading became much easier. Today he is a happy, productive person. Changing his visual habits helped dissolve his misperception that "double vision is normal for me and means I am dumb." When we become aware of visual habits, it is *then* that we can go through the vision re-education process. Dissolving misperceptions about past experiences is a very effective way to see in the present moment.

I have found that a very important milestone seems to be when a person receives the first pair of glasses. Many times this event coincides with some traumatic experience or one that was *perceived* as traumatic. The experience might have been related to a learning situation in school or a move from one city to another or an abusive relationship with someone. No matter what the circumstances, *people may freeze their vision because they do not want to see or feel what is happening around them.*

One of the first questions I ask is: "What was happening around you when you started wearing glasses? What were your experiences, thoughts, and feelings at that time?" These questions are valuable because I have found that many vision difficulties have an emotional component that needs to be addressed as part of the vision therapy process. I also ask if the person had a choice in receiving these glasses, or were they just imposed. I believe that many times glasses are prescribed as a "quick fix" to address the parent/teacher frustration of what to do with the child.

Two people who were on one of my retreats shared their stories:

Heidi is a young woman in her mid-30s who received her first pair of nearsighted glasses at age 6. "I was just beginning to learn to read, but I had great difficulty in understanding what I needed to do. I believe I had a visual coordination problem, because all the print seemed very confusing. My very intellectual father was adamant about my learning how to read. The message was: *reading is being successful.* I began to strain and tense to read, to please my father and my teachers. I became very afraid of getting the wrong answer and failing.

"One day I noticed I couldn't see the blackboard any more. This is when I went for my first pair of glasses. Over the years the more I read, the thicker my glasses became. When I wore my glasses I felt nobody could hurt me. Today I feel so ashamed about how thick my glasses are. I put them on and see so much detail. It feels like so much work. I feel helpless."

Julio, a farsighted 43-year-old man, told how he was given a prescription for glasses after he and his family moved to a new city when he was 10 years old. "I had a terribly difficult time adjusting to a new school and new friends. My parents both worked so I had no one to tell about my loneliness. I used to stay in my room and just think about the future."

Heidi's and Julio's experiences are unique to them, yet the circumstances around their first pair of glasses have much in common. The emotional aspect of how they feel about their vision is still with each of them many years after the initial events.

The next aspect in reversing deterioration of your vision starts with the question: "*Why* do you want to improve your eyesight and vision?" This is a very important question. The answer gives the vision therapist direction on how to proceed. For example, a person in one workshop answered: "Because my glasses block what I'm feeling. I want to feel myself and be free. When I wear my glasses I feel restricted." In this case, a good place to start would be with the emotional component of vision.

Another patient, who was nearsighted, said: "The muscles in my eyes are tight. I want to exercise them so they move easier." This person would probably respond well to physical activities like eye stretch and palming, and a physical/visual coordination exercise.

Below is a list of other questions I like to ask before a person starts the process of vision improvement. My recommendation to the reader is: answer each question by writing for at least 5 minutes on each topic. The purpose is to begin to bring to conscious awareness your attitudes, habits, and belief systems about your vision.

1. What has been your relationship with your eye doctor? How do you feel about your eye doctor?
2. What are your basic fears? How do these fears affect what you don't want to see?
3. How does your present vision hinder you?

4. What benefits do you get from seeing with your present vision?
5. What was your early experience in learning how to read?
6. What is your relationship with your glasses or contact lenses?
7. Describe your parents' vision.

Now you've done some of your personal groundwork. It's also important to understand some of the more common visual conditions. The physical descriptions are based on the scientific/medical model.

At the first appointment, I use three basic tests to measure the physical vision. The first involves measuring the refractive error by determining where the light bends on the retina. The second is a dynamic near-focusing test. I measure how efficiently and quickly a person can pick up a visual target, and how well the focusing response can be maintained. This test tells me how much effort a person uses when focusing to read. The third test, called the Van Orden Star, is a drawing the person does through a binocular scope. This measures how the eyes work together and how they "see" visual space. I am looking for how well a person's eyes focus together in the three-dimensional world. The drawing represents a photograph of how efficiently the eyes, brain, and body are integrated. Throughout the vision therapy, these three tests are repeated to monitor change.

In addition to the physical descriptions outlined below, I have also included the emotional/psychological/spiritual descriptions. These are based on the clinical experiences of patients I have observed and on my own vision improvement process. Using this information about some of the most common visual conditions, explore what visual condition you might have. See if you can begin to put together some of the underlying factors of why you see in a certain way.

MYOPIA (NEARSIGHTEDNESS)

Physical—In the physical form the eyeball has stretched or elongated front to back. Optically, when light enters the eye, it focuses in front of the retina. A nearsighted (minus or negative) lens is used to focus the light onto the retina, mostly onto the macula or center.

Emotional—Myopia can be seeing through a fear filter. It is an insecurity in oneself, so in compensation there is straining and trying harder. Myopia is about not trusting what one sees. It is being frozen in past perceptions. Also, one who has myopia over -3.00 diopters has often experienced some form of child abuse.

Psychological—Myopia is a pulling in of one's vision: "I can see well near, but I can't see far." The blur at a distance often makes one feel out of control. Myopia is about being more critical, analytical, judgmental, detail-oriented, linear. It is a specific and general contraction of the eyes, brain, and body. There may be an unconscious numbing-out. Since the lens used to compensate for myopia creates a virtual (unreal) image optically, one can feel unreal. The negative lens can cause one to *feel* negative. This lens focuses most of the light onto the macula alone, which deprives one of having equal distribution of light on the retina. As more equal light is distributed, more of the brain will be stimulated.

In North America, 162 million people wear corrective lenses. **One hundred million are nearsighted!**

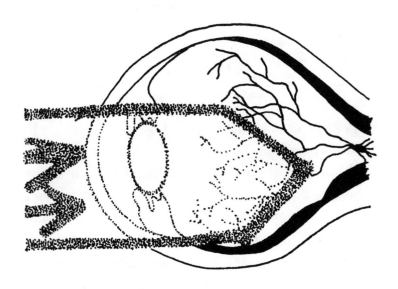

MYOPIA

Illustration by Michelle Goodman

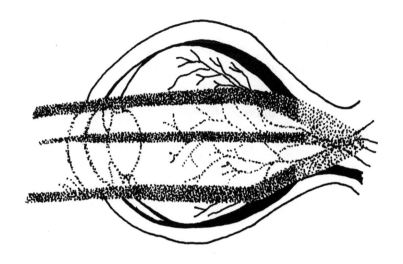

HYPEROPIA

Illustration by Michelle Goodman

HYPEROPIA (FARSIGHTEDNESS)

Physical—In the physical form the eyeball has become smaller. Optically, when light enters the eye, it focuses behind the retina. A farsighted (plus or positive) lens is used to focus the light onto the retina.

Emotional—Hyperopia can be the expression of seeing through an anger filter. It is about fearing the present so there is a tendency to put the attention into the future.

Psychological—Hyperopes can see well far away but have difficulty focusing close-up. They usually don't like crowded places. In relationships they tend to push the world away from themselves. They may also be the abusers in relationships.

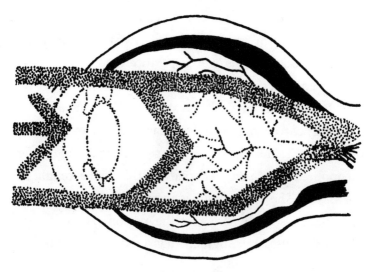

ASTIGMATISM

Illustration by Michelle Goodman

ASTIGMATISM

Physical—In the physical form the eyeball becomes egg-shaped or elliptical. Optically, when light enters the eye, part of the light focuses in front of, and part of it behind, the retina. A specific astigmatic lens is needed to focus the light onto the retina. In terms of the visual field, picture a clock: if the 12 to 6 meridian (the vertical) is showing the astigmatism, then the vertical aspect of vision will be more blurred than the rest of the visual field.

Elliot Forrest, O.D., a Behavioral Optometrist, found that a relationship exists between eye movements, head movement, posture, and visual scanning.[11] If, for example, a person's job as a computer operator requires eye scanning in the horizontal meridian, the restriction or the ignoring of the vertical scan causes the astigmatism in that restricted meridian.

Astigmatism can also be due to a twisting of the spine, pelvis, or neck. In terms of body posture, there is a tightness or restriction in the musculature.

Psychoemotional—This aspect of astigmatism can be the result of receiving mixed messages from parents and/ or teachers. That is, the father may send one message while the mother sends a different one and the child is caught in the middle. The conditioning is about going back and forth and this causes a twisting of the person. The outward distortion caused by astigmatism is a reflection of a distortion of the inner self.

PRESBYOPIA

Physical—In the physical form there is difficulty focusing at close distance. Many times this near vision begins to deteriorate around age 40. Optically, the lens and the muscles of the eye have lost some of their flexibility. To compensate for this lack of flexibility, a farsighted (plus) lens is used to refocus the light onto the retina. However, the lens only supports the disconnection to the eyes. A person becomes more dependent on the reading lens, basically losing connection with the eyes.

Psychoemotional—Not only is the visual flexibility in focusing lost, but also the emotional and the mental flexibility as well. Usually, people are avoiding focusing-in or being present with themselves. There is fear of intimacy, which is why they push their world out and away from themselves.

MACULAR DEGENERATION

Physical—In the physical form some visual acuity (central vision) is lost because the macula has become either too wet or too dried out. When one looks, there is a blurred spot in the center of the vision, which can be very bothersome if trying to drive a car or read a book.

Psychoemotional—In macular degeneration there can be a fear of losing independence. One loses the central theme in life, isn't able to focus and follow through, and has lost intention. As the central vision deteriorates, the fear may cause the peripheral vision (which is usually healthy) to close down. A person with macular degeneration often loses the wider perspective in life.

AMBLYOPIA (LAZY EYE)

Physical—There are several types of lazy eye. If there is a disease process, the amblyopia is organic in nature and the disease should be addressed before any vision therapy is done. In functional amblyopia, there is usually a decrease in visual acuity of that eye, as well as a lack of visual coordination between the eyes.

Psychoemotional—A lazy eye is one that is shut down. Many times the brain actually suppresses one of the eyes due to the interference or conflict of the eyes working so differently.

My clinical observation is that the lazy eye has been undernourished. There is a lack of stimulation because light is not being absorbed into the eye. Usually there exists unconscious fear and anger with the lazy eye.

STRABISMUS (Crossed-eye: eye turn in; Wall-eye: eye turn out; Vertical split: eye turn up or down)

Physical—In the physical form the two eyes do not work together as a team. The causes are many. Illness, accidents, stress, and heredity are factors.

The functional problem is that usually a person has not learned to control the eye muscles. This leads to double vision or to the brain's response to double vision—suppression of one of the eyes. This can affect depth perception, concentration, and hand-eye coordination.

Psychoemotional—With strabismus there exists a cosmetic aspect—how the eyes look to others. This can cause social, emotional, and self-esteem problems.

In crossed eyes (*esotropia*) there are usually issues with rigidity and inflexibility and a pulling inward, away from the world. It is a tight way of seeing.

In wall-eyes (*exotropia*) the issues have to do with not being able to focus-in. There is ability to see the whole picture but difficulty with detail. This type of vision can be very creative, but there is difficulty making decisions and following through with an action. There is usually fear about intimacy and closeness in relationships.

If the eyes break apart vertically (one eye turns up or down) there can be a split in how one sees oneself. This person usually can see both points of view, but has difficulty making a decision.

GLAUCOMA

Physical—This disease causes an increase in the pressure inside the eyeball. It can be due to poor circulation of the fluids in and out of the eye. The causes can be heredity, physical defects of the eye, stress, and other eye disease.

Psychoemotional—Usually there is a constriction in spiritual vision, often fear-based in origin. The person has pushed his or her feelings way down inside, which creates a pressure build up. In Chinese acupuncture this is known as liver energy stagnation.

CATARACTS

Physical—This is a hardening of the lens of the eye. Because of a fluid imbalance in the eye, the lens loses its transparency and becomes cloudy or opaque. When this happens, the light is blocked and visual acuity is decreased. Some causes of cataracts are diabetes, chemical imbalances in the eye from poor nutritional habits, high levels of ultraviolet exposure, stress, and heredity.

Psychoemotional—There may exist a cloudiness and uncertainty of inner vision, and a fear to look out onto life.

RETINITIS PIGMENTOSA

Physical—In a retinal condition the peripheral vision (the rods of the retina) begins to deteriorate.

Psychoemotional—Usually there is a fear of the future. There can also be a resignation in life.

CORNEAL CONDITIONS

Physical—The cornea is the transparent window at the front of the eye. There are genetic and environmental factors that can cause a clouding of the cornea.

Psychoemotional—The cornea represents the power of the eye. There is a loss of empowerment.

Some diseases of the cornea include:

PTERYGIUM: This a growth that extends from the internal part of the connective tissue of the eye to the cornea. It is a degenerative process caused by irritation from the wind or dust. Pterygiums are very common in the southwestern part of the United States.

KERATOCONUS: This condition is a thinning and stretching of the central tissue of the cornea.

VITREOUS CONDITIONS

Physical—The vitreous is the gel-like substance in the back part of the eye. Chemical and nutritional imbalances can cause changes in the vitreous.

Psychoemotional—The issue is a lack of stability for the person.

Some conditions of the vitreous include the following:

VITREOUS DETACHMENT: The vitreous separates from its attachments due to degeneration or inflammation.

VITREOUS FLOATERS: The vitreous liquifies due to shrinkage, inflammation, or chemical imbalances in the eye. Opacities such as floaters form and move freely in front of the line of vision.

RETINAL DETACHMENT

Physical—The eyeball changes shape, which causes the retina to stretch until it breaks. Stretching can occur with high degrees of myopia. This stretching can cause retinal holes or an unraveling of the retinal lining.

Psychoemotional—There can be unresolved grief, sadness, and pain. Often there is separation from the self, not wanting to focus within.

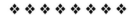

Think of your glasses as an onion. You are beginning to peel these filters (lenses) away as if you are peeling off the layers of an onion. *It is important to give yourself time to process your perceptions as you remove each layer.* If you try to speed this process, you will only create *more* stress for yourself. Go slowly, for if you try to go too fast you may miss some insight or awareness along the way. Going slowly builds a stronger foundation for healing. Take some deep breaths and relax for a few moments before going on to the next section.

VISUAL SKILLS AS A WAY OF LIFE

I have described vision as more than the ability to see 20/20 on a distance acuity chart. Below is a list of common visual skills that involve vision as a more holistic process:

1. **Eye movements**—Sometimes referred to as visual tracking, this is about moving the eyes smoothly and accurately together. This skill is very important for reading. If one loses the place, needs to keep the place using a finger, or constantly needs to re-read in order to comprehend what is being read, there is an eye movement difficulty.

2. **Focusing**—Focusing involves how we control the muscles in the eye. One skill is being able to focus clearly up close (about 14") and sustain that focus. Another is being able to effortlessly focus from near to far and back to near. Focusing involves how we control the muscles in the eye. It also involves our ability to focus the mind, body, and eyes together. This is called concentration.

There are two types of concentration: exclusive and inclusive. Exclusive refers to being focused on one point while ignoring everything else in the visual field. This takes a lot of effort and is very stressful. Inclusive involves being aware both of the self (i.e., breathing and body awareness) and of surroundings while focused on the task. This type of concentration is effortless.

People with focusing difficulties will fall asleep after a short period of reading. They may also have blurred near vision.

I like to work with the idea that focusing does not mean having to force or try harder. Focus is expansion; focus is presence.

3. **Visual Coordination**—Our eyes are meant to work as partners. They need to be similar (not the same) and integrated. If the eyes do not work together, one might either suppress (shut down) one eye or see double. Many hyperactive children see double, but this condition goes undetected. Many people think that seeing double is the way it is supposed to be. Double vision creates tremendous stress on the nervous system and confusion within the person.

When the eyes don't work together, one doesn't experience depth perception: the world is seen as flat. Yet the better the depth perception, the more proficient one will be at solving problems in school, on the job, and in relationships. As visual coordination improves, the depth perception becomes greater. Visual coordination is a very important skill that shouldn't be overlooked.

4. **Hand/Eye/Body Coordination**—This skill is a combination of the vision and motor systems. Hand/eye coordination is expressed in catching a ball, in copying from the blackboard, in handwriting. If eye movements are jerky or erratic, the hands and body also make jerky or erratic movements. It is very important that the vision and motor systems work together in a flexible, integrated way.

For example, the volleyball player spiking the winning shot, the basketball player passing the ball, the football player's defensive skills, all require finely coordinated hand/eye/body systems. Both consistency in performance and performance under pressure near the end of a game can be improved by enhancing this motor skill.

5. **Form Perception**—Form perception is becoming aware of the visual differences of shapes, objects, or words. This is a skill that can be retrained beautifully through vision therapy. One's eyes may be pointing at an object, but the mind is somewhere else, so one doesn't register what is seen. Or, there can be a mis-naming of similar objects or a misspelling of words that are similar.

6. **Bilateral Integration**—In this skill, both sides of the body are coordinated in a unified fashion. This can relate to integration of the eyes, of the brain hemispheres, or of the body. When there is a lack of bilateral integration, there will be reversals of words and letters, and of directional concepts (right, left, forward, backward). Dyslexia is the catch-all term used to label these reversal difficulties and to categorize a learning disability.

Dyslexia means confusion. It is about a lack of coordination and communication between both sides of the body, both hemispheres of the brain, and both of the eyes. Information is usually processed with one side of the body only. Dyslexia is caused by stress, emotional blocks, and to a lesser extent, an organic or a physical deficit in the brain function or by heredity. The number of true dyslexics in the population is about 8 percent, much lower than those so labeled. Vision therapy is a wonderful way to reprogram and retrain integration between the eyes, the brain, and the body.

7. **Visualization/Visual Memory**—In the experience of vision, there are three stages. The first involves taking in information through the eyes. The second involves processing the information in the brain. The third is making use of the information. Visual memory has to do with the second stage, the processing of visual input—how one makes and stores visual pictures of what is seen. The more efficient and effortless the input is, the more powerful the visual memory is. It is important for spelling, for following directions, for math, and for meditation. It is a skill that can be readily enhanced through vision therapy.

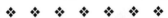

Before you move on to the next chapter, which involves your vision exercises, please consider this: you may have had learning difficulties in school or coordination problems in sports due to inefficient vision. It does not have anything to do with your intelligence quotient! You can work on your vision, so that learning, sports, and life can become happier, easier, and more peaceful.

Now that you have a basic understanding of how your personal vision works, it is time to move into ways of improving your vision.

CHAPTER FOUR

VISION ENHANCEMENT FOR DAILY LIVING

"When I SEE, suddenly I am all eyes."[12]
—Frederick Franck

Our vision has a powerful influence on our lives. It helps shape who we are in the world. Vision is a learned process based on how we experience and interact with the environment, and because we are bombarded and besieged by our world our vision can be adversely affected. It is possible to change our vision process in order to see differently.

Remember, in school, asking the teacher to SHOW us how to do something? Researchers have shown that up to 90 percent of the data we receive is through our eyes. The familiar expression, "a picture is worth a thousand words," is a reminder of that flash through our eyes.

Vision is a dynamic system. It involves not only the eyes but also the brain and body. When we move, much of our balance and orientation comes from the interaction between our peripheral vision and body coordination. When we hear or touch something, we must be able to develop an integration between these senses and our vision. The challenge is for this integrated organization of our body to be relaxed and free in order to act and choose a direction. Vision helps guide us in our movement through space.

Current statistics show that 90 percent of people in the United States will begin to wear glasses at some point in their lives. These glasses are called compensating lenses because they "provide" 20/20 sight. What they really do is treat the symptoms by correcting for blur and masking the imbalances in vision. Glasses are crutches that cause our eyes to lose flexibility. Using them, we lose control of our own eyes and vision. We become dependent on these glasses, which only represent inefficient visual habits. *Our eyes are like any other part of the body; if we exercise them they will stay young and flexible.*

Vision enhancement involves different activities and games that help one relearn how to use vision in a natural and effortless way, thus reducing the need for glasses. The sets of activities are in a menu format, and are designed so they build on each other in a balanced way. As an example, the following list shows the correlation between specific types of exercises and the visual and body coordination skills that can be improved.

EXERCISE	IMPROVEMENT
Peripheral Vision	Movement/Balance
Visual Coordination	Depth Perception Ability
Visual Focus	Concentration
Eye Movement Control	Tracking When Reading
Visualization/ Visual Memory	Learning, Following Directions
Bilateral Integration	Overcoming Dyslexic Patterns
Hand-Eye Coordination	Sports, Handwriting

In chapter 3, I described different types of visual conditions so that you can self-analyze your personal vision. The physical and personality characteristics may give you some references for your starting point for improvement. As you begin your vision enhancement program, you will bring your own vision and perceptions to each activity. These activities work in two ways: to help you reduce your need for glasses *and* to help you learn about your awareness.

The program is laid out in a 4-week plan. Practice should be 15 to 20 minutes every day. I liked doing my exercises early in the morning. This helped me begin each day by seeing the world with more clarity.

There are 3 *simple keys* for success.

1. Know specifically what you want and why you want it. Write down your specific goals in your journal as a brainstorming exercise.

2. Follow through and take action toward your goals.

3. Become an expert at observing yourself.

The exercises will help you realize how your glasses and your vision are based on past programming and conditioning. By becoming aware of old perceptions, you will begin seeing with fresh eyes moment by moment and let go of past filters. You will develop increased sensitivity toward yourself and others.

Remember, this is not about getting something right or perfect, but for you to get to know your true self, your essence. So, let's begin.

FOUR-WEEK PLAN

WEEK ONE

You are going to start with the physical aspects of seeing. The first activity involves practice at stretching your eye muscles as a way to reconnect yourself to your eyes. Experience how you hold the tension in your eyes in the midst of "doing" in the world AND REMEMBER TO BREATHE.

THUMB ROTATIONS

PURPOSE: To develop the awareness of moving your eyes in a relaxed and effortless manner.

EQUIPMENT: Your thumb

DIRECTIONS: Stand erect in a relaxed posture, one eye covered with one hand. Your other hand is thrust out—elbow straight, fingers gently clenched, and thumb erect—held directly in front of your nose. Pick out a shape (it could be a window, a picture, a lampshade, etc.) and begin to trace the outline of the shape. Follow your thumbnail with your eye, remembering to blink and breathe. After you have traced the shape in one direction, trace the shape in the opposite direction. Feel your eye muscles stretching. When you have completed this exercise, repeat for the other eye.

TIME: 2 minutes per eye

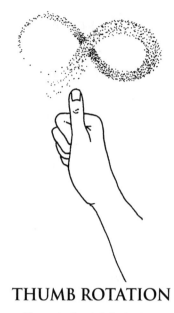

THUMB ROTATION

Illustration by Michelle Goodman

THUMB ROTATION LAZY EIGHTS

PURPOSE: Same as page 81.

EQUIPMENT: Your thumb

DIRECTIONS: Stand erect in a relaxed posture with both eyes open. Thrust your left arm out with your thumb in an erect position so it is centered between the two eyes. Start moving the left hand in a counterclockwise direction. Move your thumb up, over, and around, and back to the beginning in a lazy eight shape. (Make an infinity sign with your thumb.) After 4 rotations repeat with the right hand. Relax your body while making the lazy eight. Make the movement large enough to fill your visual field. This activity will help improve balance, centering, and coordination.

TIME: 3 minutes

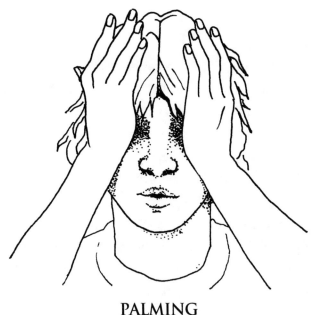

PALMING

PALMING

PURPOSE: To reduce dependency on glasses by relaxing the eyes through palming. (This exercise was developed by Dr. William Bates in the 1930s.)

EQUIPMENT: Your hands

DIRECTIONS: Palming is an excellent way to rest and refresh your eyes and mind. First, warm your hands by rubbing them together briskly. Then place your softly cupped hands over your *closed* eyes, with the heels of your hands over your eyes but not actually touching the eyelids. To keep your neck and back straight while your shoulders stay relaxed, raise your elbows to shoulder level and rest them on a stack of books or a table in front of you. As you breathe, slowly inhaling and exhaling, feel the warmth and darkness soothe your eye muscles and your whole body.

BREATH IS LIFE

Since many people forget to breathe when they use their vision, I have found that it is important to cultivate and understand the breath. Conscious breathing helps us to be in the present moment. When we are in the present moment healing takes place.

Many spiritual disciplines discuss the subject of breath. The one practice I have used which has helped me to understand my breathing is called the Mother's Breath. Below is a description of the practice. It is important that it is done exactly as it is written. The description here is taken directly from Reshad Feild's book *Here to Heal*.[13]

BREATHING PRACTICE OR THE MOTHER'S BREATH

METHOD: Sit in a hard-backed chair, feet flat on the floor, with heels together and toes apart forming a triangle. Legs should be uncrossed. Arms should be relaxed and if possible in an unstressed position; hands should rest on knees. The solar plexus has two subsidiary centres which are located in the knees. The knees are highly sensitive instruments. If you focus your attention on your knees while blindfolded, you can sense that the knees send out a beam of energy. You will not walk into a wall due to the inner sense that comes from the area of your knees.

Keeping your back straight, without forcing it, will allow the flow of energy to move as it should. With practice your back will straighten naturally. Do this exercise for about ten minutes and no longer. It can be done several times a day with safety.

Before you start the conscious breathing exercise, visualise the most beautiful object in nature you can imagine. It could be a plant, a tree, a waterfall, the sea, or whatever means something real to you. All of these practices are to help us to see God's beauty and to help us live beautiful lives.

For this practice, the eyes can be open or closed. Either way, focus on a point approximately eight feet in front of you. If your eyes are closed then put the picture of whatever you've chosen eight feet in front of you through visualisation. If you are focusing on an object, put it as close to eight feet from you as you can. *Do not meditate on a candle in this practice.* This is very important. The object of the visualisation is to help you focus your attention, not to meditate on the object itself.

Now we come to this sacred rhythm, this 7-1-7-1-7 rhythm, about which I have spoken in former books and which I have been teaching for so long. The rhythm came from ancient Egypt and there are many hieroglyphics showing how this practice, and others, are done. The method is simple though initially it may seem difficult since we are used to just breathing without any form of attention or consciousness. You may notice that the rhythm corresponds exactly to the octave in music.

First, find a point in the centre of your solar plexus area, and also a point in the centre of the chest, which we call the Heart Centre. You are going to breathe into the solar plexus, and then radiate out breath from the heart.

Please remember in working with the 7-1-7-1-7 that it is not the speed that counts, be it slow or relatively fast. It is the actual number of counts that we are talking about. Choose the speed that suits you. Breathe into the solar plexus. As you breathe, bring in all the elements of the earth, the minerals (you can even breathe in vitamins by choice if you wish!) and fill yourself with all that the body and its subtle counterparts need. Do not be embarrassed about taking what you need in the understanding that all this is done in the name of service.

Having breathed in for the count of seven, pause for one count and at the same time, bring your attention to the centre of the chest. Then breathe out for the count of seven. As you breathe out, radiate love and goodwill to all mankind from the centre of the chest, as if you are a lighthouse for the ships that are entering the harbour. Be sure to radiate not just in front of you, but also behind, and in all the six directions. At this point, there is a tremendous sense of wonder and gratitude in the realisation that, indeed, we are able to serve our fellow human beings and the planet itself.

We can choose the quality of the air that we breathe. As you progress in the practice, through correct visualisation, you can breathe the air that is circulating in certain sacred areas of the planet. You can breathe the air in Jerusalem, or Glastonbury, without leaving the chair upon which you are sitting.

The last step in the exercise, which, after all, is an alchemical process, is the refining of the breath. Begin taking only as much breath as you actually need and are given. This should require as little effort as the fluttering of a butterfly's wings. There is no more need to force the breath. In a sense, at this stage, you are not breathing. Rather, you are being breathed. Breath is Life! This is the still point in a waiting world.

To complete the practice, return to the senses. As in other practices, feel your body and take responsibility for it once more. Be awake to the room or the surroundings and finally agree that you have fulfilled what you set out to do.

EYE DIALOGUE

PURPOSE: To help you become aware of the unconscious filters you bring into your present day vision, this activity works on the deeper aspects of your vision.

EQUIPMENT: Eye patch

Journal

DIRECTIONS:

Day One

Eat a meal with one eye patched. Really observe yourself as you eat. Do not watch TV, read, or talk while you are eating. Observe your thoughts, feelings, and perceptions while you eat, and write down your discoveries. Repeat with the other eye patched.

Day Two

Take a walk outside, patching each eye alternately and notice yourself in the process.

Day Three

Spend 10 minutes looking into a mirror with each eye. Notice how you see yourself with each eye.

Day Four

Spend 10 minutes observing with each eye. Write answers to the following questions in your journal:

1. How old does each eye feel?
2. Ask your right eye how it feels about your left eye. Ask your left eye how it feels about your right eye.
3. What do you feel in your body as you have these eye conversations?
4. Are you afraid of blindness?

5. How do you feel about your eye doctors?

6. How do you feel about learning, reading, and school?

7. Left eye patched: How do you feel about your father? Right eye patched: How do you feel about your mother?

Day Five

Draw, paint, play an instrument, or sing with each eye patched separately. Notice your degree of self-expression with each eye.

Day Six

Be in communication with a trusted friend, companion, or lover for 10 minutes with each eye alternately patched. Notice how you relate with each eye, and get feedback from your partner about your behavior with each eye.

Day Seven

Spend the day thinking and feeling about your eyes working together. They are, after all, in an intimate relationship. See if your newfound awareness helps resolve the conflict between your eyes on an inner vision level.

FLASHLIGHT BALL

PURPOSE: To improve eye movement flexibility and hand-eye coordination.

EQUIPMENT:
Rubber ball
(baseball size)
and a string
*(Screw an eye
hook into the ball
and attach the string.)*
Eye patch
Flashlight

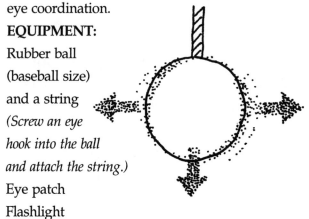

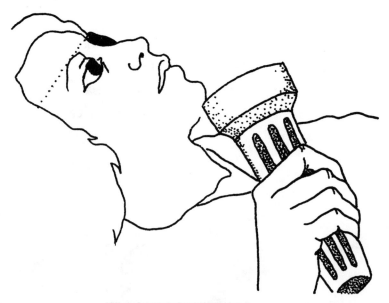

FLASHLIGHT BALL

Illustration by Michelle Goodman

DIRECTIONS: This exercise is done with glasses off. The room should be dimly lit. Hang the ball from the ceiling to within two feet of the floor. Lie on your back with the ball hanging above your chin. Patch the left eye, swing the ball from side to side, and use either hand to shine the flashlight on the swinging ball. Swing the ball horizontally, vertically, obliquely, clockwise, and counterclockwise. Keep your eye and the light on the ball as you feel your breathing and your body on the floor. Repeat with the right eye patched. This visual game works well to expand eye movements.

It is important when you do this activity to feel your eyes moving, to be aware of both the ball (central vision) and what surrounds the ball (peripheral vision), and to feel your body—all simultaneously.

On day 3 of this week, patch one eye and visualize two four-letter words, one word on each side of the ball. Swing the ball from left to right only and spell each word one letter at a time as the ball swings to that word. For example, if LOVE is on the left and PLAY is on the right, when the ball swings left, move your eye left following the ball and say "L"; when the ball swings right, move your eye right and say "P". Remember to keep the flashlight on the ball as you move your eye and spell each word. Repeat with the other eye patched.

Other words I like to use are: PEACE / HAPPY
PAINT / DANCE   LAUGH / EARTH   AWE / FUN
When you become an expert, spell one word forward while you spell the other one backward.

This is a great activity for children or the child within you.

BROCK STRING

PURPOSE: To encourage visual coordination between your eyes. After the first week of eye dialogue, your eyes should be well acquainted. This exercise was devised by Dr. Frederick Brock, a pioneer in the field of Optometric Vision Therapy.

EQUIPMENT: Brock String *(Thread 3 beads on a string so they are evenly spaced about 10 inches from each other. The string should be 3 to 4 feet long.)*

DIRECTIONS: This exercise is done with the glasses off. Fasten one end of the string to any convenient object at or slightly below eye level. Hold the other end between the thumb and forefinger just below the level of your nose. Holding the string taut at arm's length, look at the bead nearest to you. If your eyes are working together and aiming at the same place, you should see an "X" (two strings going into that bead and two strings leaving it). Notice if one of the strings fades out or is less clear than the other. Cover one eye to find out which eye is not working. If one of the strings fades out completely, then that eye is completely shut down. In order to see both strings simultaneously, follow this procedure: Cover one eye with an index card, then rapidly shift to cover the other one. Continue moving the card from one eye to the other, watching for the "X".

If you are looking at a bead and you see the strings converging before the bead, you have a tendency to cross your eyes and to hold reading material too close. This habit causes visual fatigue and blurred distance vision.

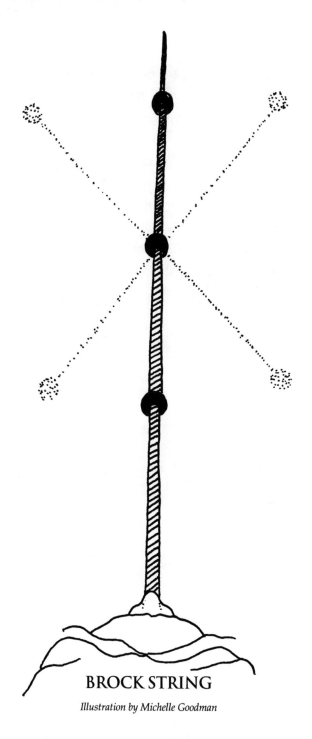

BROCK STRING

Illustration by Michelle Goodman

If you are looking at a bead and you see the intersection of the strings behind the bead, you tend to hold reading material too far away.

As improvement occurs, look at each bead and see if you can maintain an "X". Count for 3 breaths at each bead; move the "X" from bead to bead rhythmically and effortlessly. Do this exercise for 5 minutes, then palm your eyes for 30 breaths. Repeat the Brock String for 5 minutes and palm again. Notice the improvement in your visual coordination especially after palming.

CIRCLE RELAXATION: PART I

PURPOSE: To develop better integration between central and peripheral vision. When you master this exercise, you do not have separate central and peripheral visions but, in fact, have an expanded visual field. Most people are either very peripheral oriented and have difficulty focusing or they are able to focus-in but shut down peripherally.

EQUIPMENT: Circle chart *(see pages 96-97)*

DIRECTIONS: Hang the 2 circle charts at eye level next to each other on a wall. (The dots go to the outside.) Stand 6 feet from the wall. Hold your index finger 14 inches from your face centered between the circles. While looking at your finger (make sure you see only one) use peripheral vision to become aware of 3 circles. You should see a horizontal line on one, a vertical line on one, and a plus sign on the middle one. When you see 3 circles, bring your awareness to your breathing, feel yourself in your body, then take your finger away but maintain the 3 circles. After your vision is stable with the 3 circles, begin walking from side to side and forward and backward.

The object is to stay focused in visual space at about 14 inches without using your finger as a reference point, keeping the 3 circles in the peripheral vision and moving as well.

This exercise requires you to put your focus where you want it and keep it there.

When you have mastered this exercise, you have learned to create your own vision.

Although many people pay more attention to what they see outside themselves, you are learning to be connected and integrated with your inner and outer vision.

TIME: Up to 15 minutes each day

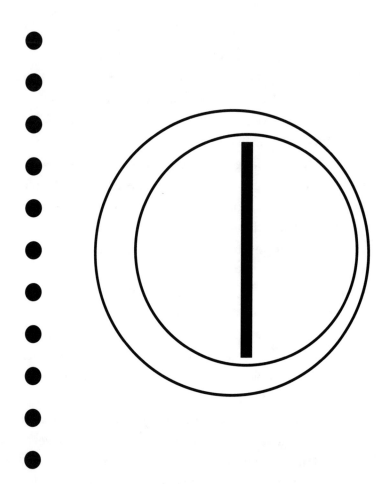

CIRCLE CHART
Duplicate and increase 135%

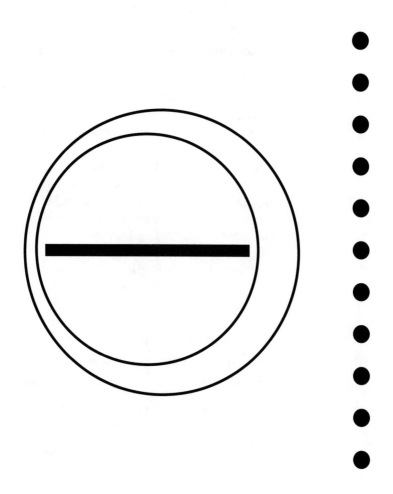

CIRCLE CHART
Duplicate and increase 135%

ANIMAL EYE CHART

PURPOSE: To stretch the eye muscles and improve movement and flexibility of eye movements.

EQUIPMENT: Animal Eye Chart

Butterfly	Freedom
Owl	Light, Magic eyes
Wildcat	Fierceness
Bear	Gentleness
Hummingbird	Multi-dimensional
Beetle	Transformation
Deer	Keenness
Badger	Fearlessness
Turtle	Purposefulness
Antelope	Agility
Eagle	Presence
Hawk	Focus

DIRECTIONS: Place your nose on the heart of the chart (the center) and begin moving your eyes upward along the path toward the butterfly. Move your eyes in a clockwise rotation along the path toward the center and then away, feeling the stretch of the muscles while blinking and breathing. If you have difficulty seeing part of the lines or an animal in a certain position, you can tilt that area of the chart away from you to see it more easily. This exercise can be done seated or standing. It can also be done with each eye separately. Each animal is associated with a certain word or words that can be used as an affirmation to help heal your vision.

TIME: 5 minutes

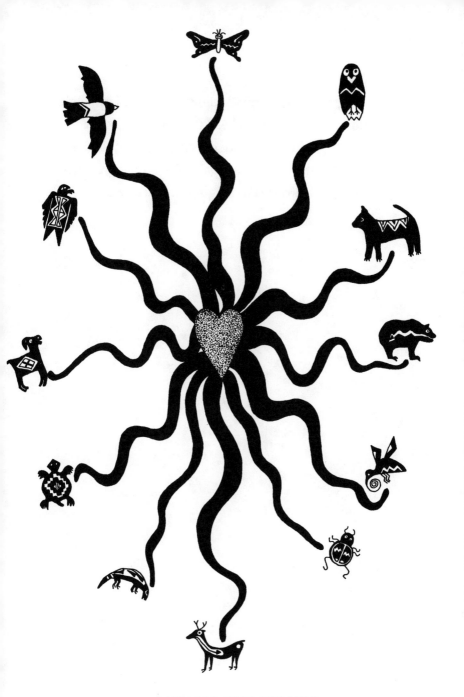

ANIMAL EYE CHART
Duplicate and increase 230%

Illustration by Michelle Goodman

BROCK STRING

Using the Brock String activity, walk in place while maintaining the "X" at each bead for 3 beats. I also recommend putting music on and dancing while doing this activity. After the 5 minutes, palm for 30 breaths, then repeat the Brock String/Palming for another cycle.

WALKING MEDITATION

PURPOSE: To develop multilateral integration of your eyes, brain, and body. This is a helpful exercise to improve concentration.

EQUIPMENT: Eye patch

DIRECTIONS: Patch your left eye. Stand in an erect posture with your feet together and arms down at your sides. You will be walking, so give yourself 6 to 8 feet of space. Raise your right arm saying, "right arm up." Then bend your knee and raise your right leg, saying, "right leg up." Move your right arm down, saying, "right arm down." Move your right leg down, putting your foot slightly ahead of the left foot, saying, "right leg down." Repeat the sequence with the left arm and left leg, moving and saying what you are doing at the same time. When you have walked this way about 6 feet, begin a different sequence (*see page 102*) while walking backward. Next, patch your right eye and say and do another sequence forward and another sequence backward.

You might use this list of sequences:

1. Right arm up
   Left leg up
   Left leg down
   Right arm down

2. Right leg up
   Right arm up
   Right leg down
   Right arm down

3. Right leg up
   Right leg down
   Right arm up
   Right arm down

4. Right leg up
   Left arm up
   Left arm down
   Right leg down

The key is to make smooth, slow movements, feel your breathing and body, and listen to yourself as you say and do the movements. The goal is to learn to experience this activity effortlessly. Notice how your mind wants to take over your wider awareness.

TIME: 5 minutes each eye

STAR RELAXATION

PURPOSE: To build on the circle relaxation by inviting you to expand your peripheral vision while focusing.

EQUIPMENT: Star Charts (*see pages 104-105*)

DIRECTIONS: In this exercise, after you see three stars as you focus at 14 inches (*see Circle Relaxation directions, page 95*), begin putting your attention on the left #1, seeing the center and right charts with your peripheral vision. This may be a challenge at first, so you might put your attention on the left part of the center star chart and then slowly move your attention to the left chart. When you are able to put your attention on the left #1 while still seeing the center and right charts, shift your attention to the center #1, then to the right #1. Return to the left chart, this time putting your attention on the #2. Then shift your attention to the center #2 and so on. When you have reached #12 on the right chart, reverse your attention from right to center to left, going from #12 back to #1. After you have mastered shifting from chart to chart, try shifting while moving from side to side. This activity will help develop more peripheral vision while focusing-in.

TIME: 15 minutes

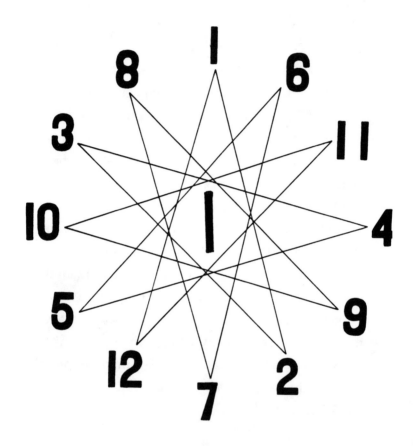

STAR CHART

Duplicate and increase 200%

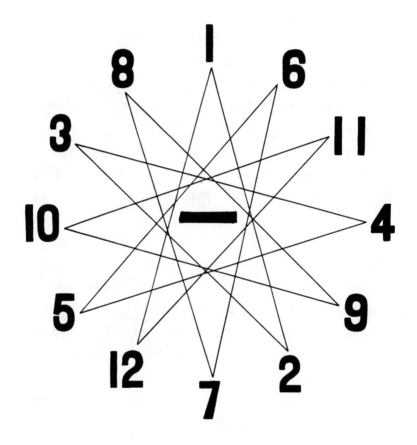

STAR CHART

Duplicate and increase 200%

NEAR-FAR FOCUS

PURPOSE: To improve flexibility in your ability to focus at different distances.

EQUIPMENT: Metronome (set at 40 beats/min.)

Two letter/number charts (*see pages 108-109*)

DIRECTIONS: This exercise is done with glasses off. Hang the chart with the large letters/numbers. Stand 6 feet away. From this distance you should be able to see the print clearly. If the print is blurry, move closer until the letters/ numbers on the chart become clear. Cover one eye with your hand and hold the small letter/number chart 14 inches in front of the uncovered eye. With the metronome beat read the first character on the chart you are holding, then shift your focus to the first character on the far chart. Read the letters and numbers back and forth from near to far, one character per beat. After you have read the entire chart, switch eyes and repeat the process. Be aware of relaxing your body and of blinking and breathing. See if you can keep the characters clear. As you get more profi- cient, move the near chart closer. When you repeat this exercise with your other eye, notice how that eye works differently.

This is a good activity to increase your visual acuity. It is excellent to retrain focusing for those people who are using reading glasses after age 40. I also use this activity with children to help them learn to copy easier and faster from the chalkboard.

TIME: This activity should be done for 5 minutes with each eye. After you complete this exercise, palm for 2 minutes before starting the next one.

```
Y L 4 B E A 8 U M H
K 2 D S U 4 L O F Z
H C 7 A E T 3 1 Y R
P B 9 G N O 5 R V T
L 2 K G B 5 U T 3 D
A W E S 8 R O X N 1
7 A P T 6 E N U R Z
V 4 R 9 S M X 2 J T
S O 2 N 6 E H U 5 W
L 8 V S P D 1 N G 7
```

LETTER / NUMBER CHART

Duplicate and increase 190%

```
Y L 4 B E A 8 U M H
K 2 D S U 4 L O F Z
H C 7 A E T 3 1 Y R
P B 9 G N O 5 R V T
L 2 K G B 5 U T 3 D
A W E S 8 R O X N 1
7 A P T 6 E N U R Z
V 4 R 9 S M X 2 J T
S O 2 N 6 E H U 5 W
L 8 V S P D 1 N G 7
```

LETTER / NUMBER CHART

109

MIND-BODY INTEGRATION

PURPOSE: To help develop whole brain integration and to retrain dyslexic patterns.

EQUIPMENT: Arrow Chart with different colored arrows
(see pages 111-112)

Metronome (set at 40 beats/min.)

DIRECTIONS: Stand 6 feet from the arrow chart, which is at eye level. Raise your arms straight in front of you, parallel to the ground. Read and do movements of level 1 through to the end of the chart, speaking and moving with the metronome beat. Go back and do each of the other levels in succession.

Level 1 Say the direction of the arrow; move your hands in the direction of the arrow.

Level 2 Alternate saying the direction of the arrow, moving your hands in the direction of the arrow, and saying the color.

Level 3 Say the direction of the arrow; move your hands in the opposite direction.

Level 4 Alternate saying the direction of the arrow and saying the color; move your hands in the opposite direction of the arrow.

Level 5 Say the opposite direction of the arrow; move your hands in the printed direction of the arrow.

Level 6 Alternate saying the opposite direction of the arrow and saying the color; move your hands in the printed direction of the arrow.

This specific exercise is powerful because you can see how you really learn and solve problems. If the linear part of the brain is used (the judgmental, critical part), the exercise cannot be done. In fact, this linear aspect of the mind actually gets in the way of performing the exercise.

This exercise is a way for you to develop awareness of when the linear mind (sometimes an aspect of mental chatter) gets in the way. "Let go" of getting the sequence right, and put forth your *intention* of what you want to do, which allows a "flow state" where the activity is effortless and you are able to let it happen. This is the intuitive part of your vision at work.

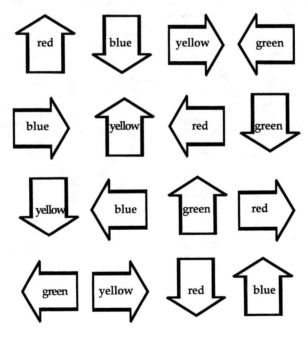

ARROW CHART
Color directions

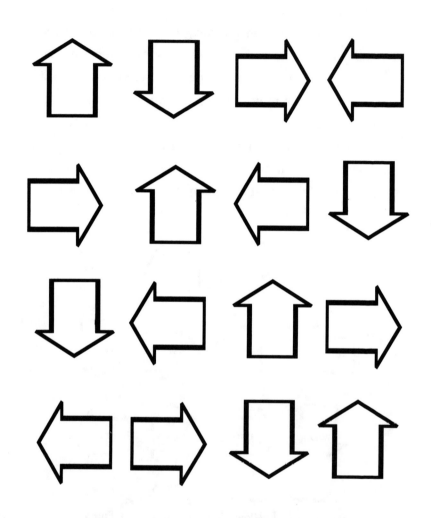

ARROW CHART
Duplicate and increase 200%.

CIRCLE RELAXATION: PART II

PURPOSE: To practice expanding peripheral vision while moving.

EQUIPMENT: Circle transparencies

(Take the circle charts provided on pages 96-97 and have them photocopied onto transparency sheets.)

Rebounder

DIRECTIONS: The transparency copies of the circles are taped to a window. The activity is done in the same manner as in Circle Relaxation: Part I. Here, however, peripheral vision involves not only side vision but also depth perception out the window. The technique is very effective for people with myopia because it helps them expand their vision into the distance while still focused at 14 inches. As you do this exercise think of expansiveness, of softness and relaxation. Vision of objects beyond the window doesn't have to be clear. Remember, the purpose of this exercise is really to help develop peripheral vision.

TIME: 15 minutes

After you have mastered this exercise standing still, try it while bouncing on a rebounder. It will be quite exhilarating!

REFERENCE WORDS
CHAPTER FIVE

KINESTHETIC: sensing the body through feeling, stimulated by body movements and tensions.

VESTIBULAR: concerning the aspect of the inner ear that affects balance and equilibrium of the brain and body.

CONVERGENCE: eyes aim slightly inward.

MULTI-HANDICAPPED: more than one of the sensory systems impaired.

VISUAL LEARNER: a person who learns best by being shown as opposed to being told.

TRAUMATIC BRAIN INJURY: trauma from a blow to the head.

FIGURE-GROUND: visual perceptual ability to see both the details and the whole picture.

VISION THERAPY AND OCCUPATIONAL THERAPY:

A MULTI-DISCIPLINARY APPROACH

*"If you can see, you can see with your nose
and smell with your ears."*[14]
—**Frederick Franck**

MULTI-HANDICAPS

Laurie is a bright, young, very alive 8 year old. She is one of my most important teachers. Every time I work with her in vision therapy, she reminds me to let go of any preconceived ideas on what she needs in the therapy process. Instead, I must rely on my intuition and creativity in order to stimulate her vision and awareness.

115

As an infant, Laurie did not roll over, creep, sit, or stand like her older sister. At 2 $\frac{1}{2}$, she was diagnosed with sensory-motor integration deficits, a left divergent strabismus (eye turning out), cortical blindness, and cerebral palsy. Luckily, her parents sought the assistance of therapists in many arenas to help stimulate Laurie in as many ways as possible. About two years ago, I met Laurie and began an intensive visual rehabilitation program. It involves visual exercises and light therapy, which was incorporated into the therapy of her occupational therapist. Laurie began to explore her environment and improve her sensory-motor integration skills.

During her sessions with me, I let Laurie "tell" me what she needed to do by observing what her nervous system wanted. In the vision therapy room, I set up 4 activities and let her choose. Activities ranged from being rolled up in a soft sponge mattress to bouncing on the large physioball or trampoline. At her present stage of vision therapy, Laurie for the first time is beginning to trust her vision to guide her in the environment. She is feeling her body!

This is one of the many cases where Optometric Vision Therapy can be used as an adjunct to other therapies in helping people with physical disabilities. One of my favorite resources in this area, *A Behavioral Vision Approach for Persons with Physical Disabilities*[15,] describes how vision therapy can be used to work with adults and children with traumatic brain injury and stroke, the multi-handicapped, and the visually impaired. Let me first speak about the process of vision in relation to these people.

Approximately 80 percent of the information that enters the eyes goes directly to the brain, where it is processed. Our other sensory processors (ears, nose, tongue, hands, feet, skin) are treated as isolated systems most of the time by medical practitioners. Working with patients, I find that the visual process shares and matches information from components of the auditory, motor, kinesthetic, and vestibular systems (the last three are important for balance and movement). I believe it is important to approach each person from a more holistic perspective, especially since the sensory and motor systems are already neurologically wired together.

Peripheral vision is intimately connected to balance and movement. It tells us about spatial relationships, depth perception, and movement. In the newborn, this aspect of vision is more highly developed than the detailed vision. As visual development evolves, an infant begins to creep and crawl, using the peripheral vision as a guide. As the child moves, visual awareness grows. The detailed or focal vision develops as a way to continually enhance the fine motor skills. If there is a limitation in either the sensory or motor aspects, mismatches begin to occur in the experiences of the child. This can cause a lag in development and growth. There is an intrinsic relationship: peripheral vision encourages movement, which stimulates the focal or detailed vision, which increases sensitivity and awareness of the environment. For eye movement to develop, there needs to be feedback from both the *kinesthetic* and *vestibular* systems.

The central peripheral vision relationship is dependent on movement and balance; any interruption in this interaction leads to adaptations by the brain that can develop into visual distortions such as myopia, hyperopia, strabismus/amblyopia, and accommodative/*convergence* difficulties.

Vision is the matching of time and space in our environment. Since movement is the catalyst that develops spatial relationships, the child needs to explore to see across the room, and then move across the room to understand how long it takes and how far he or she has to crawl. If the child cannot move, there cannot be a match of the auditory, kinesthetic, and vestibular senses with vision. It is precisely this interaction that allows the child to use eyes, ears, and body to interpret and understand the world while he or she is moving.

For the *multi-handicapped*, partially sighted child, there is a disruption of this developmental process. These children are unable to use their eye movements to provide information to the brain. Therefore, they aren't able to match time and space accurately or experience spatial relationships.

Testing

Standard visual tests, such as the Snellen visual acuity chart and the computer-generated visual field testing, measure the static part of vision. They don't give accurate information on the dynamic flow of input, processing, and output of visual information. (There are other acuity tests, but I want to limit this discussion to more functional, practical, and simple methods of visual testing.)

Observation of behavior is the best method to assess the visual capacity of a person. I observe the interactions between multi-handicapped persons and their environment. For example, when they sit on the floor or a chair, do they move or look around? Do they move or tilt their heads when looking? Are they responsive to their environment or to any outside stimulation? Many times, I will do the evaluation while a child is lying on his or her back as this seems to be the safest position. The child feels more comfortable, natural, and safe. I can observe the truest and most accurate response of a child in this position.

I use different types and sizes of light sources from penlights to flashlights to observe responsiveness to light. I usually use a light to get some kind of fixation and visual tracking response and will note the area of gaze and how long the child may fixate. I check for eye alignment to see if the eyes move together at all, and I look for some type of pupil constriction when the light is close to the face. I observe the pupil size and reaction to light; if the pupils are large (over 6mm), they are not able to focus easily.

I am very interested in whether there is any response from the peripheral vision to a target, a light, or a sound. Perhaps the child hears the sound before looking, or feels the object before moving his or her eyes to the target. I measure objectively if any lens prescription is needed and assess eye health.

I observe how fast or slow reaction is and how long focus can be sustained. I may roll children on the floor or have them jump on the trampoline while I hold their hands.

Even with multi-handicapped children, I look for any kind of visual response. I find that most multi-handicapped people are:

- ❖ very creative
- ❖ very intuitive
- ❖ independent
- ❖ holistic
- ❖ spiritual
- ❖ right-brain leading
- ❖ *visual learners*, yet usually nonvisual

First and foremost, they need acceptance and unconditional love. They need to be validated where they are. I tend to focus on the vision they do have and work in vision therapy to expand from there. The parents need to be helped to acknowledge that the multi-handicapped child is a gift and a teacher. These children cannot be put into a rigid belief system. By working with them, the healer will learn about creativity and letting go.

Therapy

When I work with multi-handicapped children, I keep many activities at my fingertips in the therapy room. Activities such as colored flashlight, ring toss, and physioball rolling integrate vision with movement—kinesthetic, vestibular, and auditory.

These children experience these activities by grasping or reaching, making a funny face, laughing, or showing eye contact with the exercise. I may repeat certain activities as a way to strengthen a specific ability. Sometimes I make a task a little more challenging to push a child to find new ways of performing the activity. I may disrupt them by using an eye patch, different prism glasses, or filters, so I can find visual input. In all of this, my intention is to turn on the switch of vision.

Many times I will move the child's body through space to help stimulate the peripheral vision. I observe what the nervous system wants to do, that is, what the body feels most comfortable doing. I balance my intention with what that body wants to do.

I offer these children fun, freedom, validation, and unconditional love. If I try to impose my belief system on them, the therapy will be hard, stressful, and ineffective. When my attitude is, "What can these children teach me?" the therapy is very effective. The goal is to blend what I want and what they need for optimal stimulation. I am acting as their guide in this process.

Activities

Below is a list of exercises and activities that are effective tools in stimulating vision for the multi-handicapped. *(See the resources list at the end of the book for address and phone number to order specific items.)*

Colored Flashlight: Cut 3" x 8" strips of the 6 colored theatrical gels to make 7 colors: red, orange, yellow, green, turquoise (blue and green), blue, and violet. Put each color in succession over the eyes and shine a flashlight or pen-light on it, so the child can see the color easily. I use the same sequence every time I do this activity to help the child develop some organizational perceptual ability. If the child is verbal at all, ask what color is seen. I spend 30 seconds to 5 minutes, depending on the attention span, having the child look through each gel. The exercise helps open up the energy in the body, brain, and eyes.

Visual Tracking: The child lies on his or her back. Above the eyes is a moving colored target, small fixation light, or a rubber ball that hangs from the ceiling. I may move the target closer, then farther from the child or change illumination in the room to stimulate visual fixation, eye movements, and central-peripheral visual organization.

Ring Toss: Encourage the child to crawl and put each ring on a colored peg.

Beanbag Toss: With the child sitting, give him or her a beanbag and show how to throw it in a nearby open-mouthed milk jug. I vary the position of the milk jug so the child can experience the visual world from all sides.

Joint Compression: *Very gently* at each joint of the body, especially the ankles, knees, and elbows, pull the joints apart, then push them closer together, about 4 to 5 times at each joint. This technique is used by massage therapists to help balance the autonomic nervous system. It works well for hyperactive children.

Mattress Roll: Have the child lie on a very soft sponge mattress, hands and arms to the sides and head above the edge of the mattress. Have the child roll up in the mattress like a jelly roll or an enchilada. The mattress acts as a container for the child to express and feel his or her body. It is relaxing and helps a child feel quiet.

Physioball Rolling: This is a 2-foot diameter ball used by occupational therapists. The child sits or lies on his or her back or stomach on the ball. The healer can roll the child over the ball. This activity works well to develop body awareness.

Trampoline (Rebounder): I have a special truck tire inner tube with mesh over it, great for a child to lie on or to jump on like a trampoline. If a child is strong enough, we hold hands and I help him or her jump on the trampoline, an activity that helps children feel their bodies. They love the aerobic workout.

Spinning/Rocking: Some children may be spun in a chair (slowly) from side to side or rocked in a rocking chair. Children who are able to walk easily can push a small rolling chair around the therapy room. These movements help stimulate the vestibular system, which encourages eye movements and low-level binocular vision.

Finger Writing: Have a child draw out different shapes and letters with his or her fingers.

Space Rugs: This activity involves a sheet with different colors, shapes, and letters printed on it. The sheet is spread out and the child is asked to put arms, legs, and other parts of the body on the different symbols. This helps children learn to focus and move their eyes with their bodies. This skill helps develop better eye-body coordination, which is very important in sports.

Overall, it is very important for these children to feel their bodies while using their vision. *Movement stimulates vision!*

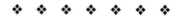

There are also other tools for stimulating the visual system:

Eye Patches: I use eye patches as a way to give each eye its own stimulation, up to 5 minutes for each eye. Using an eye patch is another way to disrupt or break up an imbedded visual pattern.

Yoked Prisms: These are special prism glasses used by many Behavioral Optometrists to help stimulate and change the spatial relationships of their patients. The prisms are used short term during an activity to stimulate and enhance peripheral vision and balance.

Weighted Vest: I have the children wear this 5-pound vest to help them feel their bodies while they are using their vision.

In general, working with the multi-handicapped, visually impaired, and learning disabled, I am less result-oriented, more process-oriented. I use three tests (pre- and post-therapy) to measure change:

1. Visual tracking (using a target)
2. Visual focusing (near-far shift in fixation)
3. Eye alignment (binocular vision)

TRAUMATIC BRAIN INJURY

In a 1990 article[16] I wrote about the use of vision therapy for *traumatic brain injury* patients. My research was collected over a five-year period while serving as a consultant with rehab centers and for occupational and speech therapists.

There were many common symptoms these people experienced. After an accident their vision showed:

1. Eyes in a divergent (posturing out) state. The eyes were more divergent focusing close-up than far away.
2. Difficulty focusing especially close-up, which led to problems while reading.
3. Memory and concentration difficulties.
4. Double vision.
5. Poor balance, coordination, and posture.
6. A loss of visual perceptual abilities.

Testing

As in the multi-handicapped population, tests for visual acuity and eye health, including a neurological examination, are important. There needs to be a functional assessment of the visual processing skills such as tracking, focusing, and eye teaming, and visual battery tests that include visual memory, spatial relationships, *figure-ground*, and visual-motor integration. Observation of behavior is the best method for measuring the functional aspects of vision. For example, if a person can walk, I observe how easily he or she moves across the room. Do both sides of the body work together? What is the balance like? What is the head and body posture when the person reads or moves the eyes? Recognizing these behaviors helps me gear the therapy activities to the functional needs of the person. If I can give some information to the occupational therapist about the person's visual system, their work can be more specific and ultimately more effective.

Therapy

When I work with traumatic brain injured patients, I like to invite their other therapists to the office to observe what I'm doing with the patient. This gives them a better understanding of how vision fits in with speech-auditory, movement, and psychoemotional aspects. I like to give occupational therapists on-going visual activities that they can incorporate into their own therapies. Generally, I will see the patient twice a month and also prescribe visual activities the occupational therapist can incorporate into the patient's daily routine. Getting all of those who work with the traumatic brain injured person to "think vision" in a therapeutic way really speeds up the rehabilitation process. When a person practices the *new* way of seeing on a daily basis, he or she is practicing and reinforcing very effective vision re-education!

Activities

Below is a list of exercises and activities that are important for improving the vision of the traumatic brain injured.

Colored Flashlight: Cut 3" x 8" strips of the 6 colored

theatrical gels: red, orange, yellow, green, turquoise (blue and green), blue, and violet. Starting with the turquoise, I put these gels over the eyes and shine the flashlight or penlight so the person can see the color easily. I use this treatment up to 20 minutes on a daily basis. I start with the turquoise color because it relaxes the person's nervous system and allows the body to come into better balance. After using this treatment regimen for 2 weeks, I begin using all 7 colors. As the person looks at each one, I ask what color they see, how they feel about it, and what it reminds them of. I spend up to 5 minutes with each color, depending on the person's attention span. The exercise helps open up the energy in the body, the brain, and the eyes.

Visual Tracking: Wearing an eye patch, the person lies on his or her back on the floor. Above the eyes is a rubber ball hanging from the ceiling (*see page 90*). Swing the ball very gently and have the person's eyes follow the swing of the ball. Swing it horizontally, vertically, obliquely, and in clockwise and counterclockwise rotation. I use an eye patch to allow each eye to move freely and independently of the other. I may move the ball closer, then farther from the person or change illumination in the room to stimulate visual fixation, visual focusing, and central-peripheral visual organization.

Letter Saccadics: The person is seated at a table. A chart of letters (*see page 129*) is placed approximately at reading distance (14"-16"). Use an eye patch and a metronome set at 40 beats per minute. The person reads the first letter on the left, then the first letter on the right at a speed of one letter per beat. After reading the outer pair of letters, he or she reads the next pair of letters on each side until reaching the middle. The second and subsequent rows follow the same sequence. After reading the whole letter chart, the person reads the outer two letters on the left column (top and bottom) and again works his or her way to the middle. He or she should continue with the next column over, following the same sequence. After the entire chart is read, have the person patch the other eye. Starting on the bottom row this time, the person reads the middle letter, then the next pair of letters, one on either side. He or she continues to read a pair of letters working out from the middle of the row, then reads the next row up, following the same sequence. After the entire chart is read, the person looks at the center letters on the right column. After reading the center pair of letters, he or she reads the next outer pair of letters and continues the sequence until the entire chart is read.

It is important to remind the person to blink and breathe while reading the chart. The goal is to be able to read the chart while moving the eyes effortlessly and efficiently. When this task becomes easy, another way to read the chart is to read the pair of letters saying the letter closest to "A" or to "Z" first and then the other letter. This added feature enhances peripheral vision and visual reaction time. Remember, read one letter per beat of the metronome. The purpose of the metronome is to train the person to become more aware of their time perception.

```
O F N P V D T C H E
Y B A K O E Z L R X
E T H W F M B K A P
B X F R T O S M V C
R A D V S X P E T O
M P O E A N C B K F
C R G D B K E P M A
F X P S M A R D L G
T M U A X S O G P B
H O S N C T K U Z L
```

LETTER CHART

Duplicate and increase 175%

Angels in the Snow: The person wears a patch over the left eye and lies on the floor with the feet together and the arms down to the side. He or she moves one limb at a time to the beat of the metronome (set at 40 beats per minute).

For example, a directional set could be, "Move the right arm (keeping it straight and along the floor) to a count of 4 beats." The person counts out loud while moving the arm in 4 equal, connected, smooth movements. The person should have their arm over their head on the fourth beat. Then the person moves the arm back to the side with 4 equal beats. The fourth beat is simultaneous with the arm reaching the side of the body.

The therapist can vary the count from 4 to 8 beats while having the patient move one limb at a time. After working with one eye for five minutes, do the same sequence with the other eye for five minutes.

After using this regimen for a minimum of 2 weeks, the patient can move 2 limbs simultaneously. The goal is to work up to all 4 limbs simultaneously. The purpose of this exercise is to develop better body awareness, bilateral integration, and effortless concentration. The metronome helps develop a more accurate time perception.

Parquetry Design

Purpose: To develop better problem-solving skills using visual perception.

Equipment: 7 pieces (Discovery Toys) and/or Parquetry Blocks (Educational Teaching Aids)

Visual perception is being able to bring meaning to what a person sees. There are many components. Visual memory is the ability to remember what is seen. Visual discrimination is the ability to see similarities and differences of objects. Parts-to-whole relationships use the ability to see both the details and the whole picture and be able to work back and forth.

These skills enhance a person's ability to use visual perception easily. The block designs require mastery at solving problems using spontaneity, intuition, and creativity. Does a person have to get stuck in the conditioning of, "I can't do it."? Can he or she just be an observer of the conditioning, continuing to see possibilities on how to solve the puzzle? The puzzles can be done with both eyes or with one eye patched.

Arrow Chart *(see Vision Exercises, pages 110-112)*
Brock String *(see Vision Exercises, pages 52 and 92-94)*

Other tools I use are yoked prisms, the weighted vest, and binasal tapes. The binasal tapes are placed on the nasal part of both lenses. The outer edge of the tape is placed where the iris (the colored part of the eye) and the sclera (the white part of the eye) meet. The tapes, also known as binasal occluders, stimulate peripheral vision, encourage simultaneous vision between the eyes, and expand the relationship to space. They are used to disrupt the normal visual pattern.

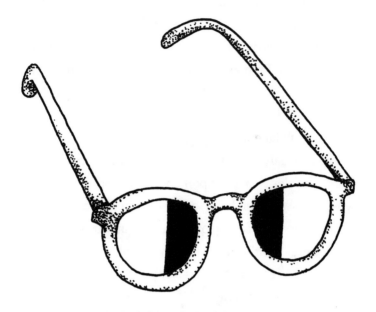

BINASAL OCCLUDERS

Illustration by Michelle Goodman

A person who has had a traumatic brain injury faces a long period of rehabilitation. Traumatic brain injury tends to bring out deeply embedded imbalances. The injury is an opportunity to heal these imbalances, to become stronger than before the injury.

REFERENCE WORDS
CHAPTER SIX

ATTENTION DEFICIT DISORDER: label describing a child who has difficulty with focus and concentration.

LEARNING DISABILITY: label describing a person's learning style that does not match the way he or she is being taught.

DEVELOPMENTAL LENSES: glasses that are pre-scribed by Behavioral Optometrists to support and nurture an immature vision system (also called learning lenses).

VISION AND LEARNING

"The way of seeing is a way of knowing."[17]
—Frederick Franck

Marcy is a creative 12 year old not performing to her potential. Her mother feels something is holding her back from really doing well in school. Marcy knows *how* to read, she is just slow at it. She skips words, loses her place, and gets tired after ten minutes of homework.

Josh is a vivacious 8 year old who was labeled with attention deficit disorder by the school psychologist. He has difficulty organizing his thoughts when he tries to write his book reports. He scored one year ahead on a standardized mathematics test administered in school, but he writes above or below the line. He is easily distracted in school and has social problems relating to his peers.

Marsha is a 20-year-old college student. She is studying to become a marine biologist. She wants to work with dolphins. She is taking the science curriculum at the local community college, but her grades are C's and D's in biology. At age 12 she was labeled dyslexic because she confused similar words when reading. She is a slow reader, and has to reread her notes many times in order to memorize the material. Her self-confidence is very low, and she feels very frustrated.

The common thread for these three young people is that they suffered some kind of vision-related learning problem. They all passed the distance visual acuity test (in my office), which measures how one sees a 1/3" letter at 20 feet. They all had difficulties with tracking, focusing, and visual coordination, aspects of vision that help a person take in information, process it in the brain, and later express it in the world.

All three of these students would be categorized as having a learning disability. In fact, they all had a hidden vision imbalance that affected reading and learning. Statistics show that 25 percent of school-age children suffer some kind of vision imbalance. Many of these problems go undetected by the conventional school vision screening. This percentage is even higher in special education classes.

Stanley Kaseno, a Behavioral Optometrist from California, has proven that there is a *strong* correlation between undiagnosed vision problems, academic nonachievement, and juvenile delinquency.[18] The tragedy is that teachers and parents are not educated about visual problems. If a child can be diagnosed in kindergarten before he or she experiences the negative feelings, conflict, and failure, much of the struggle could be avoided.

The vision difficulties children experience are caused by many factors. Vision is a learned skill. A child learns to use vision by interacting with the environment through movement. That is why creeping and crawling are very important milestones in a child's development. If there is a childhood trauma or sickness, a lag in development can occur in the visual, auditory, vestibular, kinesthetic, or motor systems. Sometimes if the in-utero or birthing experience is not normal, there can be a lag in development of any of the information gathering systems, including vision.

On average, a child's vision system does not fully develop until age 12. An overload with schoolwork in primary grades can stress the vision system and cause a breakdown in the visual skills of the child.

Not all learning difficulties are visually related. Some are language, nutritional, chemical, psychological, and motor-based problems. Behavioral Optometry can be the missing link that helps address a learning difficulty using a multi-disciplinary approach.

Richard is a 10 year old who suffers from headaches in the afternoon and his performance in school has slipped. He is no longer in the highest reading group and his grades have gone from B's to C's in spelling and math. His evaluation showed that Richard's eye focus breaks apart when he attempts to move them together. He also focuses much more with his right eye than his left eye. Much of

Richard's headaches and tension come from the effort of just trying to see the print of his books.

Instead of Richard being free to use his energy for creativity and higher degrees of problem solving, he must put his attention on trying to keep the print clear enough to read. This continuous stress interferes with the learning process.

There seems to be a higher incidence of learning disabilities and child illiteracy over the past fifteen years. In the United States, when a child falls two years or more behind in reading and writing, he or she is legally classified as learning disabled. Dr. Alan Cott says that there are about 10 million children who suffer some type of learning disability.[19] Yet, there is still the push in most schools (and by many parents) to read earlier, to get better grades, to succeed, to produce more results, to perform.

In our culture, putting a name to a problem gives us the idea we have fixed it. *Attention deficit disorder* (ADD) and *learning disabilities* (LD) are catch-all labels used by educators, psychologists, physicians, and parents who are often at a loss to discover what is really wrong. However, the labels often stick and the children become the limitations of their labels. The labels do not tell us what is really going on within the child.

What are some probable reasons for these perceived difficulties? Perhaps children actually learn differently than the way they are taught. Perhaps a child's visual system is not ready to begin reading at age 6. Instead of teaching reading at this age, suppose we allowed intuitive, creative expression, and offered more movement in the classroom. Perhaps we need to reduce the importance of grades, of excelling, of being product-oriented until a child reaches age 12. Perhaps the true art of teaching is watching how each child can absorb and learn.

Two other areas needing our particular attention are special education classes and dyslexia. In the special education classes, we need to have a more comprehensive visual screening, and to incorporate some visual activities in the classroom to improve visual processing abilities of these children. There are many children in these classes who can see the 20/20 distance acuity chart but have difficulties with visual skills such as tracking, focusing, and visual coordination. Many of these vision imbalances go undetected and the special education classrooms become nothing more than dumping grounds filled with children who aren't learning disabled at all. They have a learning style that doesn't conform to the school's method of teaching. Incorporating some vision exercises that involve visual tracking, eye-body coordination, visual memory, and spatial relationship puzzles to stimulate vision, movement, intuition, and creativity would go a long way to make learning and reading more productive and positive experiences.

Dyslexia, which means confusion in reading, involves a difficulty with the brain in terms of sequencing information. Children labeled dyslexic often experience word and letter reversal. There can be mirror writing (writing letters backwards) and a general confusion with right/left, up/down, forward/backward.

In an exciting 1986 study, using a computerized testing process, Dr. George Pavlideis[20] showed that "dyslexic" preschoolers showed irregular eye movements. Since vision therapy works with the sensory, motor, and neuromuscular systems—improving the visual tracking and visual sequencing skills—it can be an effective tool for working with children labeled dyslexic.

Vision therapy is not a substitute for education. The purpose of vision therapy is to remove the interference so that tutoring, remedial education, counseling, and occupational therapy can be more effective and lasting.

Tim is a fourth grader who was reading on a second grade level. He confused his right from left and reversed his b's and d's. He could not concentrate for more than 5 minutes at a time, and the frustration he and his parents were experiencing was painful. Tim had been tested by the school and labeled learning disabled.

During his visual evaluation, I discovered that Tim could only follow a moving target with his eyes by moving his whole head. When he tried to only move his eyes, the quality of the movement was erratic and jerky. He also could not use both sides of his body together, only one side at a time. Being able to tell Tim that he had a specific vision imbalance that was interfering with learning, and that he could do something to eliminate the problem, provided much relief to him and his parents.

After two months of vision therapy, Tim brought his reading up one grade level. Also, his grades improved to B's and A's, and he began to play baseball. The dyslexia pattern was significantly reduced. It is important to know that not all dyslexia patterns are reduced as fast as in Tim's case. However, if you or your child has learning difficulties or has been labeled with dyslexia or attention deficit disorder, at least have his or her vision system evaluated by a Behavioral Optometrist. Every bit helps!

Our society is a long way from agreement on this question, but we can ask, "How much do attitude and self-esteem affect learning?" My experience is that they are very important. Children need a lot of love, support, nurturing, and positive experiences to feel like they belong in the world.

It is important for teachers, resource room specialists, psychologists, guidance counselors, school nurses, and physicians to make a connection between observable behaviors and vision problems. Below is a list of some things to look for:

Physical symptoms
1. Red, sore, or tired eyes
2. Excessive blinking, eye rubbing, or squinting
3. Closing one eye or tilting the head when reading
4. Complaints of blurred or double vision
5. An eye turning in or out; erratic and jerky eye movements
6. Sensitivity to sunlight or fluorescent lighting

Behaviors

1. Losing the place or continually rereading words or sentences
2. Skipping lines, writing numbers in the wrong columns
3. Needing to mark the place with a finger
4. Avoiding close-up work
5. Holding books close when reading
6. Writing with face close to the page
7. Easily distracted
8. Reporting double vision
9. Writing or printing very slowly
10. Difficulty with writing on ruled lines
11. Avoiding eye-hand coordination activities such as tying laces, catching, batting
12. Difficulty copying from chalkboard
13. Confusing left and right
14. Difficulty with organizing space on a paper
15. Transposing on/no, saw/was, 6/9
16. Not working to potential
17. Low self-esteem
18. Short attention span
19. Irritability
20. Daydreaming
21. Fatigue, frustration, stress

Once the vision imbalance is detected, parents should find a Behavioral Optometrist who can test the skills of vision, which are:

1. Eye tracking
2. Focusing
3. Visual coordination
4. Hand-eye coordination
5. Visual perceptual skills, including
   - ❖ visual memory
   - ❖ form perception
   - ❖ spatial relationships
   - ❖ central-peripheral visual organization
   - ❖ visual motor integration
   - ❖ bilateral integration

Developmental (low plus) *lenses* can be used as a tool to help a child focus, to use peripheral vision more easily, and to process visual information with more efficiency. The lenses are prescribed based on a dynamic focusing test (the child reads or focuses on a moving target and the doctor measures flexibility and response to the focusing by placing different preventive lenses over the eyes). These learning lenses allow more light into the eyes, which stimulates more of the retina and brain. They help retrain the visual system to see *more* with less effort, and are worn generally six months to a year while the child is doing vision therapy. After the child begins to become visually efficient with the lenses, in many cases they won't be needed anymore.

If there are vision imbalances, vision therapy is a wonderful treatment to help the child reeducate eyes, brain, and body to work together and process information more easily and with less stress. Depending on the severity of the visual difficulty, the therapy lasts an average of three to six months of weekly 45-minute sessions.

Children today seem to be experiencing more and more breakdown in their visual skills. One of the reasons is the amount of television a child watches every day. Television is a very passive experience. It programs us to sit in a trance-like state, discouraging any kind of creative problem solving. Children need a variety of experiences in order to develop fully. Stimulating vision requires movement, creative thinking, and self-awareness. One way to encourage healthy vision development is to limit the amount of television watched.

Another aspect for enhancing proper vision development has to do with what we eat. Generally if a child can avoid foods with refined sugar and artificial flavors, and has only a small amount of dairy products, the eyes and the vision will remain clear and healthy. *(See chapter 9 for more information on nutrition and vision.)*

The third factor essential for ensuring a healthy vision system is to have your preschool-age child tested by a Behavioral Optometrist before vision imbalances occur. Researchers have shown that up to 80 percent of classroom learning takes place through the vision system. This is especially true in the early years of school: "Show me a funny picture, show me a square design, point to the red balloon." The earlier you can catch the problem, the easier it is to remedy it.

It is far easier to practice prevention than to use a drug to control a hyperactive child, one who may get lost in the shuffle in a special education classroom or become a learning disabled adult. Vision therapy is a wonderful tool to help children become better learners!

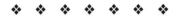

Wendy Ogden is a vision therapist in our office who closely identifies with children who have learning difficulties. An educator and counselor for the past twenty years, she holds a teaching credential in Special Education and counseling certificates in Psychosynthesis and Neural Linguistic Programming. She has also been a chiropractic assistant and has completed basic training in homeopathy, which she incorporates into her practice. For the past five years Wendy has been practicing Educational Kinesiology, a system that establishes integration and balance in the whole mind/body system.

WENDY'S STORY

Learning was always something that seemed separate from me. My earliest memory of this separateness came in first grade when I received my first report card and I had a "D" in reading and a "D" in art. I was devastated and cried for hours. My response was to avoid art forever. I forced myself to read and buried myself in novels for the rest of my school years.

I survived school because of sheer willpower. It took hours to complete homework that my friends completed easily. I was determined to never again see anything below a "B" on my report cards and through perseverance managed to earn high marks until university.

It did not occur to me that I was stupid; I just knew that for me school meant long hours. Many nights found me in tears trying to solve the mystery of "compare and contrast". Learning seemed like such a long struggle. Learning was pain.

In college I realized for the first time that I could not really express myself because analytic left brain process was beyond me. However, it did not ever occur to me that this was a problem. I "felt" my way through school and had good friends who helped me write papers.

A colleague of mine couldn't really understand that I had learning difficulties. Then one day she said to me, "I finally get it. You *are* learning disabled, but only in terms of our educational system." *This is true not only for me, but for all the children and adults who learn differently.*

Our educational system is locked behind its own door. It knows only one way to educate—left brain/analytical. It is a system that fosters inadequacy and failure in some individuals.

My interest in locked doors and unhappy children has led me to many different classes, training, and conferences. With Dr. Berne's insight, using vision training, I realized that I was a child whose first language was intuition, not English. Had I been given the keys to transforming this intuition into organized thoughts my mind would have opened. Had I had access to vision therapy as a 6 year old failing reading, my school experience might have been successful rather than a source of pain.

I did not understand the full extent of my difficulty in learning until I began doing vision therapy. I had successfully avoided areas like the hard sciences, analytical writing, and math where I was unsuccessful and stressed. I had not really explored my creative side since my "D" in art in first grade. Instead I focused on body and feeling and became a counselor. I had developed a defensive attitude toward anything demanding mental analysis.

Through vision training I began to understand that people see with the brain. The first time I heard about Dr. Berne's work I intuitively knew this was my next step. I began observing his work and doing my own vision therapy and knew I had found a missing piece, both in myself and for my clients. The vision work gave structure to my big-picture way of seeing. It allowed me to fit the pieces into the whole or break the whole into pieces and to see how they connected.

Education means "to draw forth." Vision therapy works because it attempts to draw forth the person's natural ability to see, to learn and to be whole. I now have more choice in my life and have begun to melt the frozen places in my brain, which gives me more freedom to express my core identity.

I have learned that failure is useful feedback and that mistakes are opportunities to honestly access what I need in order to move forward, to become more whole, and to have more choice in my life. It's not about getting it right or performing well so the teacher or therapist thinks I'm a really bright, intelligent, whole person. When I first started vision therapy I was very aware of the need to get a particular task right, and getting it right was more important than self-understanding. Many of my clients experience these same feelings and begin to explore how "getting it right" has limited their vision and choices and, therefore, the experiential world. It was a relief and a new beginning when I was able to experience comfortable, meaningful learning. Too much of education today focuses on results and getting it right and ignores the process of learning as pure joy and movement.

Light therapy (*see chapter 7*) can provide a profound way to touch the depths of our own essence, our own soulness. Through the light therapy, I have gained a deep experience of self-love and connectedness with myself and the universal light. The process was noninvasive, yet deeply transformative. Usually in light therapy the relationship is between the client and the light. The true therapist is the light. It was empowering to work directly with the light rather than with a therapist. I was seeing, feeling, and exploring how I block the light, how I avoid being my core self. My changes occur because I allow the light to come in and shine on the dark places so that I can see.

Vision is the umbrella because every theory we create and live by relates to our inner and outer vision. I often ask clients what having better vision will do for them; in 90 percent of the cases their responses reveal the desire for transpersonal or spiritual qualities such as freedom, inner peace, connectedness, compassion, and love. When I began hearing these responses, I knew that I had found the form of my life's work. To see with new eyes is to connect the head and the heart, the eyes and the soul.

REFERENCE WORDS
CHAPTER SEVEN

VISIBLE SPECTRUM: electromagnetic waves seen by the human eye.

ULTRAVIOLET (UV): radiation electromagnetic waves just beyond the violet vibration of the visible spectrum.

NANOMETER: unit of measure—one billionth of a meter.

LIGHT THERAPY: treatment using color to rebalance the environment within the organism.

HYPOTHALAMUS: the part of the brain that regulates metabolic processes of the body.

AUTONOMIC NERVOUS SYSTEM: part of the nervous system that governs involuntary body action such as the heartbeat, intestines, and glands.

ENDOCRINE SYSTEM: the ductless glands, which distribute secretions into the blood stream.

VISION, LIGHT THERAPY, AND OPTOMETRY

"Your eye is the lamp of the body; when your eye is sound, your whole body is full of light; but when it is not sound, your body is full of darkness."[21]

—Luke 11:34

About fifteen billion years ago, a great silent fireball exploded, precipitating the beginning of the universe. Quantum physicists have postulated that the fireball was comprised of particles of matter and energy that came together under heat and pressure to cause a powerful explosion of light. One of the most fascinating aspects of this theory is that all the particles of matter and energy that existed at the origin of the fireball are still in every part of the universe today. In other words, all the particles in our bodies had their origins from that fireball. The light from the fireball is the same light that exists in us!

The plant kingdom was the first place where miraculously, living things used light as food. In order for living things to survive and grow, they must feed off the sun. In fact, 99 percent of all organisms need sunlight as food.

Photosynthesis, the process that converts light into food in plants is initiated by chlorophyll molecules. It is chlorophyll that plants use to capture the sunlight.

When scientists began studying the retinal cells of the eye, they found the retinal membrane to have some of the same characteristics as chlorophyll molecules. Both capture the light from the sun and convert that light into a chemical impulse. Chlorophyll converts light into food. The retina converts light into an impulse that is sent to the brain, where vision takes place.

Quantum physics has proved that light is one of the core elements that supports life on Earth. Without light, there would be no life. So, the question I raise today is: Why have we suddenly developed "allergies" to light? Why this scare that sunlight is harmful to humans; that certain aspects of the non-*visible spectrum* such as *ultraviolet* cause cataracts, cancer, and so on? We are told to cover ourselves with sunscreen, wear heavy dark sunglasses, and block the light from reaching us. Doesn't this blocking out involve an alienation or separation from ourselves? Here is my theory:

As humans, we have evolved with the intelligence that has created science and technology. The advances made have been phenomenal on one level. But on a deeper level, becoming so focused on science and technology has put us out of touch with our true essence. We ignore our environment, pollute the Earth, do not pay attention to our relationships or to ourselves. *We* are becoming toxic and these toxins are causing the breakdown of our immune systems. The air, water, and food are contaminated and the light, which through the history of life has been inherent to our very existence, has become the enemy.

ULTRAVIOLET LIGHT

Some new research suggests that people need to get back into a relationship with light. Dr. John Ott, a pioneer in studying light and health, has done a number of studies on the importance of natural light on the physiology and behavior of human beings. Dr. Ott believes that, just as we need a balanced food diet, we also need a balanced light diet. He feels that ultraviolet (UV) is an important nutrient as part of the full spectrum of light just as vitamin B complex is an important nutrient as part of a multivitamin tablet.[22]

Dr. Zane Kime has found that trace amounts of UV light, given in short exposures, enhance the body's resistance to infections, decrease blood pressure, increase cardiac output, lower the resting heart rate, lower cholesterol, increase energy, endurance, and muscular strength, and cause the production of vitamin D in the body, which aids in the absorption of calcium and other minerals.[23]

In traditional mainstream studies, which perpetuate this fear of sunlight and ultraviolet radiation, massive doses of UV exposure were used on animals to create skin cancer and cataracts. Certainly great amounts of anything—

water, aspirin, heat—can cause harm but trace amounts of nutrients and minerals—and to these we add UV—are very important to maintain our bodies in balance. As Dr. Ott says, if we give too much oxygen to a baby at birth, it will go blind. Should we then avoid oxygen in our lives?

TYPES OF ULTRAVIOLET LIGHT

The energy of the sun travels as electromagnetic waves to reach the Earth. These waves are measured in *nanometers* (nm). Visible light is the part of the electromagnetic spectrum we see (a very small section); infrared and ultraviolet light are part of the invisible spectrum.

In classifying the types of UV light, there are three levels to consider. The first, UVA (320nm-380nm), causes tanning of the skin. UVB (290nm-320nm) starts the production of vitamin D and the absorption of calcium and other minerals in the body. UVC (100nm-290nm), which is filtered out by the Earth's ozone, contains properties that kill viruses and bacteria.

All three types of ultraviolet waves are necessary in trace amounts to support health and well-being. However, with the depletion of the ozone layer and our greater awareness of what is needed to take care of our immune systems, we are realizing the necessity of receiving a balanced amount of sunlight. In terms of vision care, these are some general guidelines for patients:

1. Take off your sunglasses, contact lenses, and/or glasses and spend up to one hour a day outdoors. Don't look directly at the sun but just sit or take a walk in the

natural light. Not only will you get the benefits of sunlight but your vision may improve as well. Be sensitive to yourself and if the sun feels too bright, wear a hat or sit in the shade or on a porch. The safe periods for going without sunglasses are before 10:00 am and after 4:00 pm. Native Americans say when the sun is pink (at sunrise or sunset) its rays are very healing. When the sun is white, don't look directly at it.

2. If you want to wear sunglasses, especially for skiing or water sports, buy a neutral gray lens, which cuts out the sunlight in a balanced way. Most sun lenses block all UV light. Environmental Lighting Concepts has designed full spectrum sunglasses that are a more balanced sun lens. Their sun lens transmits 40 percent of UVA and 5 percent of UVB to the eyes.

3. Don't wear contact lenses that are tinted; your eyes will receive unbalanced light. People's eyes become light-sensitive because glasses, contacts, and sunglasses block *all* UV as well as other portions of the spectrum.

Light-sensitive means that eyes are not able to process light easily and effortlessly. There is probably a vision imbalance, perhaps even a deeper imbalance in the nervous system or endocrine system.

There are people who have dilated pupils but are not taking any medications. They are usually light-sensitive, have difficulty focusing at near, and experience a high level of stress. The accelerator part of the nervous system (the sympathetic system) is working overtime as a way to adapt to the stress. The adrenal glands are producing a high level of adrenalin, and the person is feeling overwhelmed and tense. *Light therapy* is one way to reduce the stress and help restore balance to the body.

Many professionals are using tints, glare coatings, and dark lenses to treat learning disabilities and/or vision imbalances. Some tints can provide more comfort for the patients and even in some cases improve reading performance, but the tints *are not* causing deep-level changes within the patient. The tints treat symptoms only, which serves to drive the imbalance further inside.

These are general approaches for enhancing your relationship with light in an optimal way. If you have cataracts, macular degeneration, pterygiums, any eye disease, or light sensitivity, please seek the advice of your eye doctor. Remember, any changes made to open your body to light *must be done very slowly, gently, and moderately.* Let your body tell you what is appropriate for you, and if you are uncertain, seek the advice of a professional.

LIGHT AS MEDICINE

In my first year of optometry school, one of my instructors described the process of how light is refracted (bent) as it enters the eye and focuses on the retina. He stopped, however, at what happens to the light when it goes from the retina to the optic nerve and then to the brain. What happens is that 75 percent of the light that enters the eye goes to the back of the brain where the vision centers are. Twenty-five percent goes down the hypothalamic pathway to the *hypothalamus*, which is the regulator of both the *autonomic nervous system* (sympathetic and parasympathetic) and the *endocrine system*.

One part of the hypothalamus regulates the sympathetic nervous system, which increases hormonal output. The second part regulates the parasympathetic nervous system, which decreases hormonal output. As part of the central nervous system, the autonomic nervous system controls internal actions of the body such as heartbeat, breathing, and digestion. The sympathetic nervous system supports movement and action, and the parasympathetic nervous system works to rejuvenate and rebuild the body.

In terms of endocrine function, the hypothalamus both stimulates and inhibits hormonal function. It regulates the secretions of the pituitary gland, thus affecting the body's hormonal functions. The hypothalamus is in constant communication with the glands and the organs of the body.

It also regulates energy balance, growth and maturation, circulation and breathing, emotions, reproduction, heat regulation, activity, and sleep. It acts as the central conductor in controlling the life mechanisms in the body.

Another player in the regulation of the body's internal clock, one which is directly affected by light, is the pineal gland. Tucked beneath the brain, slightly above and behind the pituitary gland, this pea-size organ "turns on" every night by releasing melatonin—a hormone that helps signal the body that it is time for sleep. The pineal is directly tied into the dark/light cycle. If we work the nightshift, the body gets out of rhythm, and the dose of melatonin produced can leave us feeling depressed and lethargic.

Researchers are beginning to use light therapy introduced through the eyes to regulate the function of the nervous and endocrine systems in the body. For example, light therapy is being used as a way to turn off the pineal gland's production of melatonin to help people who work the nightshift stay fully awake. Penn State's Center for Cell Research, a NASA-funded center, and Dr. George Brainard, a neurologist of Jefferson Medical College in Philadelphia, have done a great deal of work with SAD (seasonal affective disorder) using light therapy. Scientists are only beginning to scratch the surface on how light affects our endocrine and nervous systems.

A new field focusing on energetic medicine is emerging, combining understanding of the molecular structure with energy and vibration on an auric level. Based on Einstein's theory of energy and matter, vibrational medicine views the human as having many dimensions. These layers involve energy fields that interface with the physical body. Researchers have shown how these energy fields within and surrounding the body carry information for growth, development, and repair of the physical/cellular body.

Within the genes on DNA strands, there exist both the molecular mechanisms and the subtle energy systems that govern the development of the individual cells. Researchers are now finding that many disease processes have their origins at these subtle energy levels.

Both the physical and energetic levels of humans have been described by ancient and contemporary schools of healing throughout the world. Acupuncture meridians, homeopathic remedies, herbal medicine, and Ayurvedic practices are only now being recognized by Western technology as influences on the physiology of cellular systems and vital energy of the body.

One of my most transforming experiences was beginning to contact the vital energies in my own body. I began to explore these energies through the practice of yoga and meditation in 1986. Until that time, I was totally split between my body and my mind. I relied exclusively on my intellect to process information in the world.

The practice of yoga helped me begin to unite my body, mind, and spirit into one system. The yoga postures helped me rejuvenate and relax and for the first time I began to experience the state of being-in-harmony. As my practice of yoga deepened, my body awareness also increased. I began to experience the chakras (the vital energy centers) of my body. *(See chapter 8 for a discussion of chakras.)* I discovered that this energy radiated to every cell, that it expressed itself through memories, behaviors, emotions, and actions. About this time I was introduced to the science of Syntonics, an optometric treatment utilizing different colors (energy wavelengths) of light to improve different visual conditions and overcome diseases. I was intrigued by the possibility of using energy to facilitate healing, so I began exploring its use with patients.

One of my first cases involved a 68-year-old woman who was suffering from age-related macular degeneration (ARMD). Visual acuity in her right eye (the eye that had ARMD) was 20/700. According to the Syntonic College of

Optometry, macular degeneration should be treated with 20 treatments of blue-green light. I decided to follow the treatment plan and to my surprise, her visual acuity then improved to 20/150. I didn't do any vision exercises with her; *the light therapy actually changed her vision on a physical level.*

I began to study the origins of light and color therapy and found that in ancient times solar mythology was very much a part of the culture of the Greeks, Egyptians, and Hebrews. The Egyptians, for example, developed healing temples inside a pyramid to take advantage of the universal healing properties of light and color. In Greece, Pythagoras gathered information and taught about the healing light using Egyptian teachings about soul mastery. Heliopolis, the Greek "City of the Sun", had special healing temples in which sunlight was broken down into its different colors to treat various medical conditions.

In the twentieth century, one of the first pioneers in the field of light and color healing was Dinshah P. Ghadiali. Known as "Dinshah", he received a medical education in India and later emigrated to the United States. He developed a light treatment called "Spectro-Chrome Therapy", a mathematical approach using twelve color filters, that projected light on different body parts as a way to heal various imbalances. Much of Dinshah's work was derived from an 1878 book by Dr. Edwin Babbitt,[24] which explained that sunlight filtered through colored glass, or water imbued with such colored rays, could be used to heal the body.

Dinshah's fundamental principle contained two parts: that our bodies are made up of chemical elements as well as a certain balance of color waves; and that disease occurs when a certain imbalance exists between these chemical elements and the color waves. He believed that by projecting a certain color on the body, the balance would be restored without the harmful side effects of chemical drugs. Color, of course, works on an energetic level and does not directly affect the organs. When the body's energy level was restored, the physical body would return to a state of healthful balance.

Dinshah's treatment regimen included the following: green was the equilibrator or balancer of the body; lemon (yellow-green) was considered for chronic conditions; turquoise (blue-green) for acute conditions; magenta was used for creating a deeper balance in the body; scarlet, to increase activity in the body; purple to decrease activity in the body. For any pain or bleeding in the body, indigo was used.[25]

At about the same time that Dinshah was using the "Spectro-Chrome Therapy," Dr. Harry Riley Spitler [26] began to use light and color therapy directly on the eyes. Dr. Spitler, a medical doctor as well as an optometrist, conducted research leading to our understanding that different parts of the brain are directly related to the autonomic nervous system and to the endocrine system. He also found that eyes had the most direct connection through nerve pathways to these two systems. By applying different colors of light through the eyes, Dr. Spitler could rebalance the nervous system and improve visual processing. In 1933, he founded the College of Syntonic Optometry. Today this group of practitioners is involved in the education and research of Ocular Phototherapy.

In the 1980s, Jacob Liberman, O.D., Ph.D., applied his own ideas to Syntonic Optometry. He initially used a device called a syntonizer that directs different colors (frequencies) of light into the eyes. Dr. Liberman coined the term "color allergy" to describe the state in which a person is unreceptive to a particular color. His research on light and color led to the development of an educational device called the Color Receptivity Trainer. Dr. Liberman's first book, *Light, Medicine of the Future,* is a comprehensive collection of history and research on the healing properties of light. He has had a major influence on the utilization of light and color for healing and vision.

OPTOMETRY AND LIGHT THERAPY

Early in my own practice, I began to use light and color therapy as an adjunct to vision therapy in working with patients. At first, I used Dr. Spitler's regimen from the College of Syntonic Optometry. I found that treatment with a certain frequency (color), based only on a person's visual condition, would not go deeply enough to cause core level changes in that person's visual system. There are many levels of a person's vision and of their use of awareness. Habits and conditioning can reside in the physical, emotional, psychological, and/or spiritual aspects of a person.

Success comes from being able to access most or all of these levels when working with patients.

Combining Dr. Liberman's methods with the principles of Syntonic Optometry, I found that certain colors tended to re-awaken old memories. I was using the light on myself in the same fashion, and as I continued my practice of yoga and meditation, I began to connect to different energy centers in my body.

Each frequency (color) tends to correspond to a different part of our bodies. In the process of seeing old unconscious patterns, we may re-awaken memories, emotions, or experiences that were too painful for us to look at at the time. In essence, light is a clear mirror in which we may discover ourselves in a deeper way. The fastest and most direct way to heal our outer vision is to heal the inner vision first.

In terms of our awareness, there is an outer vision— how we see the world—and an inner vision—how we see ourselves. The clearer we can see inside ourselves, without denial, the clearer our outer vision will become. Light seems to be able to cut through the roadblocks and resistances we have set up—such as ego, personality, and the rational mind—and helps us discover unconscious patterns about ourselves. It is as though light fills up all the dark places of the inner vision. When we look at light, what we see is a clear mirror of ourselves.

REFERENCE WORDS
CHAPTER EIGHT

CHAKRA: an energy center in the body.

PSYCHOSPIRITUAL: a combination of mind/body/ spirit.

PRANA: life-force energy (Sanskrit term).

TRANSFERENCE: the patient's feelings, thoughts, and wishes are transferred to the therapist.

ENERGY AND LIGHT

"This eye is my lens. This eye is the lens of the heart, open to the world."[27]
—**Frederick Franck**

CHAKRAS

The term *"chakra"* is from the Sanskrit meaning "wheel". The concept was used and written about by ancient Indian yogis and is still important to present-day practitioners. Western scientists have generally ignored these centers, but recently they have begun to see anatomical and physiological relationships to the body. For example, the position of each chakra relates directly to both a major nerve plexus and an endocrine gland.

The seven major chakras correspond to deep wisdom on the physical, emotional, psychological, and spiritual levels of a person. Each chakra links the glands, organs, and nervous system together in an integrated fashion. The more people are able to open these energy centers the better they will be able to support their own wellness. The chakras are set in a vertical column from the base of the spine to the top of the head as listed below:

CHAKRA	POSITION
1st–Root	Coccyx, base of spine
2nd–Sacral	Below the navel, near spleen
3rd–Solar Plexus	Below tip of sternum
4th–Heart Center	Directly over heart and thymus
5th–Throat	Middle of throat (over thyroid and larynx)
6th–Third Eye	Mid-forehead
7th–Crown	Top of head

Physiologically, each chakra relates to a flow of energy from the spiritual level to the cellular structure of the physical body. The energy created by the chakras effects cellular changes in the physical body.

Since the endocrine system has such a powerful influence on the central nervous system, energy from the chakras can have a deep effect on a person's physiology. Research in the field of psycho-neuroimmunology suggests a connection between these nonphysical energy vortexes, the endocrine and immune systems, and the brain.

Each chakra also has been associated with *psychospiritual* meanings in the body. When the chakras become blocked or clogged, the life-force energy (*prana*, in Sanskrit) is not available to the vitality of the physical body.

Using light and color therapy is one way to open up any blocks in the chakras. Sometimes when the chakras

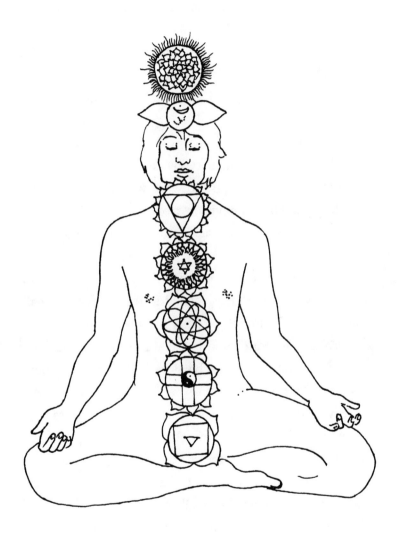

CHAKRA DIAGRAM

Illustration by Michelle Goodman

ENERGY AND LIGHT

open, old memories, emotions, and perceptions that have been stored are released as a way of detoxification. If we go deeply into our feelings with a trained therapist who can guide us in working with the light, it is possible to release these old patterns. During the light treatment, there may be a feeling of heat or a movement of energy. After the blocked energy dissipates, there can be feelings of peace and openness.

Opening these vital energy centers helps reconnect the organs, glands, and nervous centers of the body. In terms of vision, using light to work with the chakras is a way to expand the inner vision of oneself. Each of the major chakras has certain emotional and spiritual meanings associated with it.

The *root chakra* is located at the base of the spine in the coccygeal region. It is related to the colon and small intestine and is involved with the release of digestive materials. The root chakra is a place where intense fears about the will to live can be stored. In terms of vision, people with myopia tend to hold blocked unconscious energy concerning survival issues. This chakra can be where one experiences primal energy. It helps in the alignment of the rest of the chakras. The color is red.

The *sacral chakra* is located halfway between the navel and the genitals. It is related to the gonads, reproductive organs, urinary bladder, large and small intestines, and the lumbar vertebrae. From a psychospiritual perspective, this chakra is the expression of passion, vibrancy, and sensuality. It is a blending of the masculine and feminine energies within. When this chakra is blocked there is a conflict in one's sexuality, which shows up as pain, grief, shame. A blocked chakra can be due to unresolved sexual abuse. With the vision, one eye usually sees more clearly than the other eye. There can be significant myopia or hyperopia present (over 3 diopters). The color is orange.

The *solar plexus chakra* is located above the navel and below the ribs. It provides energy to the stomach, gall bladder, spleen, liver, and pancreas. From a psychospiritual perspective, this chakra relates to the ability to access personal power. It is the center of the will, the intellectual power, and the ego. Often when the solar plexus chakra is blocked, it is a result of inner anger, of feeling like a victim, or of disempowerment. This chakra represents the fire within oneself. Opening it can lead to connecting to the source of one's energy. In terms of vision, the person usually has major hyperopia or myopia when this chakra is blocked (over 3 diopters). Many times the power of the person resides in his or her lenses—the focus is outside of the self. This results in a deep insecurity about seeing, trusting, and loving intimately in relationship. The color is yellow.

The *heart center chakra* is located over the heart and the thymus gland. This chakra supports the heart, lungs, breasts, and circulatory system. On a psychospiritual level, the heart chakra represents the expression of love and compassion, the love that fosters goodwill, forgiveness, nurturance, and detachment. Self-love is very important to opening the heart chakra. On a vision level, when this chakra is blocked the person has either pushed the visual world away, or pulled the world very close in. The person is seeing through a fear filter. Glaucoma can also result from a blockage of this chakra. The color is green.

The *throat center chakra* is located in the middle of the throat. On the physical level, this chakra influences the parathyroid and thyroid glands, the vocal chords, the mouth, the trachea, and cervical vertebrae. It can also influence the vagus nerve, which travels from the brainstem to the heart, via the neck. The vagus nerve is responsible for regulating the parasympathetic nervous system. On a psychospiritual level, the throat chakra involves communication and self-expression. When this chakra is blocked, there is a difficulty with creative expression. On a vision level, myopia results when the person does not express true inner feelings or inner needs. It is fear that closes down the throat chakra and causes a narrow view. The color turquoise, which opens the throat chakra, is especially effective when working with people to reduce myopia. The color is blue.

The *brow or third eye chakra* is located in the middle of the forehead. On a physical level, this chakra influences the sinuses, the eyes, the pineal organ, and the pituitary gland. Psychospiritually, this chakra represents the ability to see one's destiny. When the third eye chakra is open, it helps connect one's intuition with the universal consciousness. The third eye chakra is also involved with being able to see one's inner vision, which is being connected to spirit. The more clearly one sees his or her spirit, the more clearly one's essence can express in the world. An energy blockage in this chakra can result in endocrine imbalances, sinus problems, and mental confusion. In terms of vision, the two eyes not working together will interfere with the effectiveness of the third eye chakra. The color is indigo.

The *crown chakra* is located at the top of the head. On a physical level, the crown chakra influences the nervous system, the cerebral cortex, and the integration between the right and left hemispheres of the brain. On a psychospiritual level this chakra represents the aspect of oneself that involves higher states of awareness and a deep spiritual knowing of oneself and the outer world. When this chakra is open, there is a total alignment of the body, mind, and spirit of the person. When the chakra is closed, there can be confusion (which could be dyslexia) or more serious forms of mental illness. On a vision level, when the spiritual aspect of the self is opened, the person may see auras and experience a state of connection with everything in the universe. The color is purple.

Light therapy is one way to access and move chakra energy. Since each chakra has a certain color vibration, in the process of the chakra opening certain memories and emotions may feel strong and sometimes uncomfortable when the patient takes in the light through the eyes. Knowing the colors that affect certain feelings and corresponding organs in the body helps determine which color might be triggering feelings in a patient.

When I use light to work with the inner vision, my

intention is to "open up" the energy in the body, to reprogram old patterns and conditioning at a cellular vibrational level. The key here is for the patient to experience the light filling up the body. As that happens, the blocked energy may open up and the uncomfortable experience may dissipate. As the old energetic pattern is released, the patient may gain more clarity on his or her inner vision.

When I treat people with this method, they are able to discover core misperceptions about awareness and behavior. Opening up the chakras seems to give the person more space within and helps to free them more easily from their conditioning. As one becomes free from conditioning, there is an effortless trust about intuition and creativity.

The procedure works like this: The patient is seated in a dimly lit room, looking into the color machine. (I use both the College of Syntonic Optometry Syntonizer and Dr. Liberman's Color Receptivity Trainer.) I use ruby as the introductory color which starts the process. My intention is to move up the chakras and keep the energy moving up the body. I also use a flicker device, adjusting the speed of the flicker to the point that it is slightly uncomfortable for the person. The next color I show is red. The standard question I ask is, "Tell me what you see and what you feel." This procedure is repeated for orange, yellow, green, blue, indigo, and violet. As the person looks at each color, I ask him or her to tune into body awareness and report any sensations, feelings, or memories that are observed. It is very important for the patient to completely feel his or her body while looking at the colors.

As a facilitator of this process, I keep asking questions, then mirroring the response. Sometimes to help a person focus, I ask what they would like to get out of the session. I reinforce that they are in charge and if they want to stop at any time, or if they do not want to talk about certain aspects of themselves, they have that choice. The light machine is a very effective tool because it acts as a buffer between the facilitator and the patient, so *transference* is reduced. The light is available for people to discover their deepest truth.

Sometimes when a person has a lazy eye or an eye that has been deprived of stimulation, I treat the weaker eye using this method. I also may put different lenses or filters over both eyes while using the light to enhance or change the patient's processing ability.

With children, I utilize a similar approach. However, the dialoguing is much simpler than with adults. I will show each color and ask what the color reminds them of, or how they feel about the color. I may even tell a short story while they are looking at the color. The light works on reprogramming the subconscious and unconscious part of the child. Hyperactivity, word and letter reversals, double vision, blurred vision, poor tracking and focusing, have been reduced just using this method. The light therapy is an adjunct to the vision exercises. Using the light can speed up and cause breakthroughs in the process of improving vision. This type of light and visual stimulation also works well with low functioning multi-handicapped and brain injured children.

CASE HISTORIES

Of the hundreds of patients I have worked with, I have chosen a few case histories that show the usefulness of light and color therapy in the process of vision improvement.

Case History 1

Paul is a 45-year-old male who came to the office with the hope of reducing his myopia. He had been wearing corrective lenses since age 6. The prescription had been increased over the years to - 6.50 diopters in each eye. His physical health was fair. He had been suffering from the Epstein-Barr virus for the past two years and was being treated with acupuncture and herbs to improve his energy level.

For the first month of vision therapy, we concentrated more on the physical exercises such as the Animal Eye Chart, the Circle Chart, and the Brock String. We also did body awareness exercises such as Angels in the Snow and the Vision Meditation Walk. I treated Paul with the turquoise color filter, which relaxed his eyes and opened his peripheral vision. About one month into the therapy, I saw that Paul began to experience his feelings on a deeper level, so I spoke to him about the emotional aspects of his vision. He began to become aware of how numb he had made his eyes and his body. He felt that in order to reduce his dependency on glasses, he needed to go deeper than the physical level with his visual skills.

At the first light therapy session, the red triggered the feeling and memory of tightening his body and eyes to survive the abuse from his father. Although it had been 40 years since that took place, he was still carrying this reaction in his present-day nervous system. Each color in that first session seemed to be uncomfortable, but as he sat with the colors new awarenesses opened for Paul.

In the three months of vision therapy, Paul and I did four light therapy sessions together. As of this writing, Paul's prescription is - 3.50 diopters with 20/25 acuity. He wears disposable contact lenses and I have prescribed a pair of - 2.00 diopters lenses for him to continue wearing at home and for his daily practices. Paul couldn't believe how much less stress there was on his nervous system and in his body, how much more energy he had, and how much more positive he felt about his life.

Case History 2

Chris is a 6-year-old girl diagnosed by her occupational therapist with a sensory motor integration difficulty. She had a right divergent strabismus (her right eye wandered out), amblyopia (lazy eye) in that eye, and saw double when she read. She also had difficulty with handwriting, sequencing, and fine motor skills such as tying her shoes and catching a ball. She actually told me she was allergic to light. Her general health was fine and she wasn't on any medication.

With many children, it is helpful initially to work on a level that doesn't involve language or letters. The activities can be geared with body movement, spatial activities, and light, all of which improve confidence and self-esteem.

With Chris we started each session with light therapy. Sometimes I would do the light therapy with just the right lazy eye, and sometimes with both eyes together. I combined this treatment with the body integration activity called Angels in the Snow and several eye movement and eye focusing activities. In a month, Chris's divergent strabismus reduced by 40 percent. Her lazy eye improved two lines on the visual acuity chart and she was seeing almost as well as with the good eye. She only saw double when she was very tired. Her handwriting improved and her mother reported she was much happier and more at peace with herself.

In cases like this, I use the light and color as a way to open the person and the physical exercises as a way to anchor in *new* vision and awareness patterns.

Case History 3

Bill is a 4-year-old boy referred by an occupational therapist. He was diagnosed with cerebral palsy, seizures, and cortical blindness. Bill's pediatric ophthalmologist had given him the diagnosis of cortical blindness caused by brain damage suffered during a seizure. When I examined Bill, I found he had approximately 60 percent use of his peripheral vision. He showed about - 1.00 diopter of myopia in both eyes. His visual world was blurred, which is why he put his head very close to his toys when he was playing. His gross motor skills showed he could creep and crawl, and he also showed some fine motor ability with his left hand.

I immediately began using different colored gels with a flashlight to stimulate eye movements and eye focusing in different areas of gaze. Bill loved to look at the different colors, and I found that incorporating the color therapy with the visual-motor skills (tracking, focusing, and visual coordination) made a big difference in the way Bill began to process information. He began to establish eye contact with people, he began to transition independently from standing to sitting in a cube chair, and he began to stand up from his chair to reach for objects placed above him. Later in his therapy, I would hold a colored flashlight in front of him and have him push a chair across the room.

I have worked with Bill for about one year, and the teachers in his special needs school have noticed that he has better focus, more eye contact, and easier balance. Color and light therapy was the language that Bill understood. It was the key that opened up his vision.

Case History 4 *(This is Wini's story in her own words.)*

I am a 34-year-old woman who has worn lenses since the age of 12. My lens prescription had gradually increased over the years to - 3.00 diopters in both eyes. My ophthal-mologist's prognosis was that vision "just continues to get worse with age and time." I was tired of that answer. I knew there was a better way; I just hadn't found it yet.

At the age of 24, after spending 2 years enduring Western medicine's idea of curing cancer, from surgery and radiation to chemotherapy, I made a radical shift. I quit chemotherapy, moved to a new city, began acupuncture treatments, changed my diet (and eventually my entire life), and began healing. That was 10 years ago. Based on my own healing experience, I knew my ophthalmologist's prognosis was flawed. I strongly believed in the body's ability to heal and I believed that anything, no matter how severe, could shift. I also trusted that I could find the teacher I needed to help me change my vision. When two women in my women's group mentioned a new "vision therapist" had moved to town, I knew immediately he was the one and I made an appointment. Three months later, I was no longer wearing lenses.

As I write, I'm sitting on a park bench, with my 4-week-old baby next to me, looking at the trees. My visual acuity shifts as I write this account of my experience. You see, writing this, an expression of myself, is a healing experience.

Vision, I learned, has little to do with the eyes and everything to do with the heart. Vision therapy became another journey of discovery. I was able to uncover events in my past that had caused my mind to put up blocks to good vision. I learned that my body reacted to those experiences by disengaging my right eye from my left so that they no longer functioned as a team. I learned that my inner voices, established as a child, kept my spirit caged, incapable of healthy self-expression of who I am and how I feel. I chose not to see at the age of 12 because there were things in my life I couldn't bear to see. Discovering abuse in my childhood was a necessary revelation for visual healing. I began believing that it was really OK to see. Eye muscle exercises helped my left eye begin reacquaintance with my right eye so they could begin to work together again. Expressing the pain of my caged spirit began the reclamation of my creative self.

I couldn't force these things to happen, I could only allow them. To force vision with the use of lenses is to rigidly control that which must be allowed freedom to thrive. The more I allow my vision to happen, the more my heart opens. The more my heart opens, the more vision I receive. I continue to move toward more visual acuity.

The effects have been far-reaching. More and more, I allow myself to express how I feel with my husband, my sons, my friends, and myself. As my heart opens, I'm more accepting of people and the environment and am able to listen (see) more. During the course of vision therapy, I also practiced Iyengar yoga and participated in personal therapy. These things have been powerful teachers. Mind/body/ spirit integration is now my self-proclaimed prognosis.

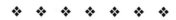

Overall, I believe that light is a very powerful tool for working on deep healing. I have found two purposes for these wonderful channels, the eyes: to receive light and to radiate light. The more we can take in, the more we can give—and giving (radiating) is an aspect of our self-expression.

REFERENCE WORDS
CHAPTER NINE

ELECTROMAGNETIC ENERGY: waves of electricity and magnetism given off by most objects.

FULL SPECTRUM LIGHT: artificial lighting that simulates sunlight.

EPITHELIAL: protective outer layer of the cornea and other surfaces of the body.

I.U.: International Units of measurement of food elements.

mg: milligrams.

COLLAGEN: the connective tissue between cells.

KERATOCONUS: thinning of the cornea, which shows as a protrusion.

NUTRITION AND VISION

"I had a vision because I was seeing in the sacred manner of the world." [28]
—**Black Elk, Sioux Indian**

The science of Ayurveda (from India) says that diet influences the mind and the mind in turn influences our choice of diet. When we eat in a balanced manner, we will be clear, peaceful, and joyful. The food that nourishes us is necessary for the whole body of course, but the eyes and the brain—comprising less than 2 percent of the total body weight—use approximately 25 percent of the body's nutrition.[29]

Eating three balanced meals a day is not enough for many people. There are biological stresses that can affect the absorption of the food we eat. Hans Selye was one of the first people who studied stress. He found that a certain amount of stress—called "eustress"—was beneficial to cause

181

change and growth. However, when the stress became too great—"distress"—it caused a breakdown in an organism's system. In today's world, we are bombarded with many different types of stress: psychological stress, allergy overload, environmental toxicity, drug side effects, radiation, electromagnetic pollution, and negative thought patterns. These bombardments affect the endocrine, nervous, and immune systems, ultimately causing disease.

Stress affects our eyes and vision in many ways. Nearpoint activities such as working at the computer or studying in school can cause visual adaptations such as myopia, hyperopia, or astigmatism as ways to compensate for inefficient and harmful habits.

Not expressing emotions can show up in the eyes as a pressure build up (glaucoma) or a cloudiness of the lens (cataracts). One of the most important aspects of stress is that it is not only the activity we are doing that causes the stress. Attitudes and thought patterns that we bring to the activity can contribute to stress and a breakdown in the body.

There are several methods to use to practice stress reduction. Relaxation techniques such as palming, meditation, progressive muscle relaxation for the mind-body, exercise, massage therapy, and yoga are effective ways to reduce levels of stress and develop inner peace. What we do nutritionally can also help in managing stress and can promote well-being.

Since nutrition is really about how we absorb and process energy whether it be in the form of light, herbs, or food, I decided to interview two women who work in the field of energy medicine and nutrition.

DR. HAZEL PARCELLS

The first woman I met with was Dr. Hazel R. Parcells, a Ph.D. and diplomate in Naturopathy, a Naturopathic Physician, a Chiropractor, and the founder of Parcells System of Scientific Living, Inc. in Albuquerque.

Dr. Parcells is 104 years old. She works every day in her clinic and is developing a center for restoring the *electromagnetic energy* of the body. Dr. Parcells believes that food poisoned by toxic additives, pollution, and radiation creates a deadly environment for humans and other living things. She teaches techniques for enhancing food absorption and digestion, as well as methods for removing toxic radiation and other pollutants from the food and from the body.

Dr. Parcells discovered the famous "Clorox treatment" to remove bacteria, fungus, pesticide and herbicide sprays, heavy metals, and other toxins from vegetables, fruits, and meats. (Foods are soaked in a bath of 1/2 teaspoon of Clorox added to one gallon of water for 15-30 minutes depending on the types of foods, then soaked in plain water for 15 minutes. According to Dr. Parcells, Clorox brand bleach should be used because of its special formulation.)

Dr. Parcells also uses full spectrum light treatments, color therapy, and cooking methods that are easy and effective. One of her principles is that the essence of life is color; that is, without color there can be no life. Dr. Parcells demonstrated this point by placing a crystal prism (which reflects all the colors of the spectrum) over a glass of distilled water. By using either the direct sunlight or a full spectrum light she can raise the energy level of the water 3600 percent (as measured by a system developed by Dr. Parcells). When we drink the water, the cells are replenished by the particular color they need. Dr. Parcells' research shows these benefits from drinking this energized water: clearing of radiation, x-rays, carbon monoxide, cobalt 60, and metallics.

Tap water can also be cleaned of harmful germs and chemicals by using *full spectrum light*. Dr. Parcells recommends filling a glass gallon jug with water, then placing it under the full spectrum lights for 1 hour. This will clear the water of any chemicals or additives.

Cobalt 60, according to Dr. Parcells, is being used to extend the shelf life of food. However, cobalt 60 kills *everything* it comes in contact with, including living tissue. Some symptoms from eating food treated with cobalt 60 include exhaustion, cramps, and attacks on any weak place in the body.

Through her research Dr. Parcells has developed an easy process to remove cobalt 60 from food. A light called the Thea-Lite is combined with a 12" x 12" green-blue normalizing unit with a strong magnetic field that neutralizes any pollutants, metallics, and spray residue found in the food. Combining this process with the Clorox bath gives the *most* energy to foods, and reduces food allergies.

In terms of deteriorating vision and eye health, Dr. Parcells believes that usually the eyes are not getting the proper amount of oxygen from the blood. The major culprit is the amount of carbon monoxide in the air we breathe. Dr. Parcells says she doesn't treat disease: "Drugs make you worse and you don't even know it." She says if people can change their environment, the body will heal naturally.

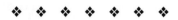

AMADEA MORNINGSTAR

The second woman I interviewed was Amadea Morningstar, a Western-trained nutritionist who incorporated Ayurvedic principles into her 20 years of private practice and classes. No longer in practice, she now writes about Ayurvedic cooking[30] and is considered an expert in her field.

As Amadea said, "In Ayurveda, fresh food is a primary key to healing. The fresher the food, the more vitality it has to share with us. Fresh food can be cooked or raw, and includes fruits, vegetables, and fresh unprocessed dairy, as well as dried beans and grains which are freshly made. A person's eyes reflect their overall energy, and how we eat has a direct connection to our vision and well-being.

"One traditional Ayurvedic way to directly enhance nourishment to the eyes might sound a little odd to us now, but it is quite helpful. Once or twice a day, on rising and before bed, a small dab of clarified butter (ghee) can be gently massaged into the nasal passages. This relieves sinus congestion, releases pent-up feeling, and often improves vision.

"How well we absorb nutrients affects eye health. Foods which are frozen, fried, or in other ways extensively processed, are harder to digest and offer less energy to us. They can also contribute to an accumulation of toxins in the body, which can cloud vision. Other foods to avoid for this same reason include refined sugar and grains and concentrated sweets."

She went on to say that there is a direct connection between liver function (where vitamin A is stored) and the eyes. Some symptoms of decreased liver function include red, strained, irritated, lusterless, or tired eyes. (In Chinese medicine, when acupuncturists treat the liver meridian, patients often report an improvement in vision.) Foods which are soothing to the liver include vitamin A-rich sweet potatoes, winter squash, broccoli, apricots, and cantaloupe. However, we need the mineral zinc to be able to release vitamin A from its storage spaces in the liver, and zinc is often in short supply in the American diet. Some rich sources of zinc include beans, pumpkin seeds, sunflower seeds, nuts, and mushrooms.

There are a number of good digestive herbal tea combinations to maximize benefits from the food we eat. Fresh ginger tea, or ginger with turmeric and fennel or coriander are useful, drunk with or following meals. These herbs, plus basil, cumin and oregano, also assist digestion when they are cooked with food. Turmeric helps to digest proteins and purify the blood.

There can be specific nutritional deficiencies which affect vision:

- ❖ Children with allergies often need more natural vitamin B complex and vitamin C to nourish the liver, respiratory, and nervous systems.
- ❖ Children diagnosed with attention deficit disorder are frequently short on the minerals calcium, magnesium, and zinc. They can have problems with blood sugar regulation or food sensitivities, which can cloud the vision. Vitamins B6 and B12 are often low.
- ❖ Children and adults with myopia are often deficient in calcium. It is thought that this deficiency may contribute to the distortion of the eye muscles and eye shape in myopia.
- ❖ Because the trace mineral chromium aids the body in getting insulin to the cells, it can be helpful to the person with vision problems related to adult-onset diabetes.

Amadea says that vision problems are usually a signal that other body systems need help in balancing as well.

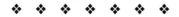

My own basic philosophy is "I eat to live." Food is a source of fuel, which gives me energy. Probably the most important ingredient put into the food I eat is love—if I am cooking, this is an act of self-love and nurturing myself.

In general, I have found the Ayurvedic philosophy useful in terms of cooking with certain foods and herbs as a way to balance my constitution. Going to an Ayurvedic physician or reading a good book on Ayurveda can give some basic guidelines on how to cook based on each individual constitution.

In terms of the eyes, there are some very effective and proven guidelines for promoting a healthy vision system. Please be advised that these are general guidelines. Seek the counsel of a professional before you make major changes in your nutrition.

Vitamin A: An oil-soluble vitamin that comes in two forms—retinol, found in animal foods, and carotene, found in plants. Vitamin A enhances healthy *epithelial* tissue throughout the body and increases the strength of the mucous membranes. It promotes a healthy cornea, conjunctiva, and retina. It can help in the reduction of burning and itching of the eyes and reduce the frequency of sties.

The mineral zinc works synergistically to make vitamin A more effective. Zinc is responsible for improving the digestive enzymes and helps increase the oxygen input to all the tissues of the eye. Researchers have found that low zinc levels along with high levels of cadmium and lead are found in children with learning-related difficulties.[31]

I have worked with a number of patients to improve their "night blindness" and the adjustment of vision when going from the dark to the light or vice versa, using 10,000 to 15,000 *I.U.* per day of Vitamin A for one month coupled with 20 to 25 *mg* of zinc per day. I have also used this vitamin therapy regimen successfully to help reduce the dry-eye syndrome many people suffer. There are special Vita-A drops that also can be used to reduce the dry-eye syndrome.

Sources of retinol include eggs, whole milk, and cheese. Sources of carotene include fresh vegetables such as parsley, carrots, turnips, lettuce, and spinach. Sources of zinc include mild, green leafy vegetables, onions, and pumpkin seeds.

Vitamin C: A water-soluble vitamin that helps promote *collagen* (connective tissue) growth between the cells and the body, aids in oxygenating the cells, and helps flush the body of any accumulated toxins. Vitamin C is valuable for maintaining a healthy sclera, lens, and cornea. Megadoses of vitamin C—5000 I.U. daily—have been used in Europe to reduce the intraocular pressure. This type of therapy is called orthomolecular medicine; physicians treat illness by using high dosages of vitamins in a pharmacological manner just as the conventional physician uses drugs to treat illness.

Sources of vitamin C include citrus fruits, melons, strawberries, leafy green vegetables, cabbage, tomatoes, and sweet vegetables (yellow and red bell peppers, yams, and zucchini).

Vitamin E: Part of the fat-soluble group that helps keep cells healthy and free from waste products known as free radicals. I recommend vitamin E for those people who have retinal degeneration because it helps remove toxins and improves the circulation between the retinal cells. I also use vitamin E to improve the circulation in the lens to reduce the formation of cataracts. Recommended dosage is 400 I.U. daily. Sources of vitamin E include green leafy vegetables, nuts, whole wheat, and eggs.

Vitamin B Complex: A series of B vitamins that promote and enhance a healthy nervous system. These vitamins work effectively to treat macular degeneration of the fovea, and also promote a healthy lens and conjunctiva. Sources include avocados, legumes, yogurt, peas, asparagus, oatmeal, cheese, almonds, mushrooms, figs, seafood, whole grains, cabbage, cantaloupe, kelp, and milk. Recommended daily dosages: B1 (thiamine mononitrate)–50 mg; B2 (riboflavin)—50 mg; B6 (pyridoxine hydrochloride)–50 mg; B12 (cyanocobalamin)–100 mg; folic acid–400 mg; biotin–400 mg; pantothenic acid–100 mg; niacinamide–300 mg.

Calcium: An inorganic element that helps support the normal growth of bones and teeth. Patients going through a stage of increased myopia or suffering from the condition of *keratoconus* have a deficiency in calcium. The recommended dosage is 800 to 1200 mg per day. Sources of calcium include raw vegetables (kale, cauliflower, dark leafy greens, broccoli), almonds, salmon, milk, and cheese.

Chromium: A trace mineral comprised of many of the hormones and enzymes found in the body. *Eating white sugar regularly depletes the body of this trace element.* Researchers have shown that a chromium deficiency increases the risk factor for developing myopia and other visual focusing difficulties.[32] The recommended dosage is 300 to 500 mg. Sources of chromium include whole grains, starchy fruits and vegetables (peaches, pears, jerusalem artichokes, potatoes), and shellfish.

Spirulina: A blue-green microalgae that is very nutritious and very healthy for the eyes and the whole body. It contains about 70 percent naturally occurring protein, beta-carotene (pro-vitamin A), B-complex vitamins, iron, magnesium, selenium, enzymes, DNA, RNA, and potassium. It is extremely digestible and is a very effective source of oxygenating the cells and increasing energy. Because spirulina is so pure and natural, it helps replenish the essential vitamins and minerals in the body. *(See Resources for an address to order spirulina.)*

There are 3 herbal extracts I would like to mention: Ginkgold, Bilberry, and *Succus Cineraria*.

Ginkgold: Dr. William Schwabe of Germany began researching the ginkgo extract from plants in the late 1950s. His research found that ginkgo helps the brain utilize the intake of oxygen in the body and works as a free radical scavenger in the cells. Ginkgo therapy can help impaired visual perception, improve mental alertness and memory, and reduce depression, anxiety, and mood instability. *(See Resources for an address to order Schwabe's Ginkgold.)*

Bilberry: This fruit extract comes from a berry that is found in Northern Europe and Asia. Clinical research has shown that the bilberry is effective in improving night vision and can accelerate the adjustment to darkness. A number of clinical studies show that this extract helps to reduce vascular disorders of the blood vessels and capillaries in the body. It can help restore balance to the blood vessel walls and slow down leaks of the membranes, and works as an anticoagulant. It is an effective herb to help control the circulation in the eyes of diabetics. It is available in 375 mg capsules.

Bilberry extract is being used widely in Europe, and has become available in pharmacies in the United States. *(See Resources for an address to order Bilberry.)*

Succus Cineraria Maritima: This extract can be used to reduce cataracts in the eye. This preparation works to increase the circulation between the tissues in the eye and provides normal metabolism, which promotes a normal physiology of the eye. A clinical study performed by ophthalmologists showed that out of 40 patients with onset of cataracts over 4 years, 22.5 percent showed a reduction of the opacity while using *succus cineraria maritima.* The most effective use of this extract is to apply it in the early stages of cataract formation. (Physician's prescription needed.)

In the desert Southwest, we are surrounded by many plants that have major medicinal qualities for healing. Two of my favorite sources on this subject are: *Los Remedios: Traditional Herbal Remedies of the Southwest* by Michael Moore and *Earth Medicine—Earth Food: Plant Remedies, Drugs, and Natural Foods of the North American Indians* by Michael A. Weiner. I specifically like to use eyewashes to treat sore, painful, or irritated eyes. It is important that any eyewash used be made fresh each time and be isotonic (the same salinity as tears). To make the water isotonic dissolve 1/4 teaspoon of salt in a cup of warm water. The eyewashes I use involve making a simple tea. This is done by putting a teaspoon of the herb in a cup. Pour a cup of boiling water over the herb and steep for 15 minutes. Strain the water through cheesecloth. For seeds or powdered herbs, use a small teaspoon; for whole leaves or twigs use a tablespoon.

Below is a list of some common herbs I have used.

(Use a fresh batch of tea for each treatment.)

1. Mesquite: This herb is a favorite among Native Americans from the Southwest. The Apaches added water to the powdered leaves and then squeezed the liquid through a cloth on the eyes. Another tribe applied the sap directly on inflamed lids. It can be used as an eyewash by making a simple tea preparation.

These three herbs were used by the Blackfoot Indians to treat sore and irritated eyes. They can be made into an eyewash using the simple tea formula.

2. Yarrow (leaves and flowers)

3. Snowberry (from leaves)

4. Horsemint (from flowers)

These herbs can also be used as an eyewash with the simple tea formula.

5. Western Ragweed

6. Blue Flax leaves

7. Pluchia leaves

8. Borraja (Borage)

9. Contrayerba (Caltrop)

10. Una de Gato (Black Locust/Cat's Claw)

11. Yerba de Sangre (Oregon Grape)

12. Rosa de Castilla (Old Fashioned Red Rose)

AFTERWORD

The path of self-realization and the attainment of goals is a long and spiraling process. *Creating Your Personal Vision* is a practice of mindful vision. The specific exercises are a reminder of how you can see *all* the time—not just during the exercise period.

As your vision improves, three aspects will surface and expand: self-observation, inner nourishment, and voluntary simplicity.

Self-observation means developing more clarity of mind. It is this clarity that allows the inner vision (inward truthfulness) to dissolve the conditioned responses. It will help us become more adept at rising above our cultural conditioning.

The second aspect to appear is the ability to nourish ourselves. This means that action and stillness will become the same. It is when we experience this unity that fulfillment occurs. Everything we need is discovered inside ourselves.

The third aspect in this spiral is voluntary simplicity. Learning to open our vision is about discovering freedom, living in harmony, and expressing our true natures. Letting go of complexity, intricacy, and artificiality encourages voluntary simplicity.

Seeing mindfully dissolves our fear and helps make it possible to live fully each moment of our life. It is matching inner vision with outer seeing.

As a wise Eskimo elder sings:
"My whole body
is covered with eyes.
Behold it.
I see all around."[33]

VISION EXERCISES FOR SPECIFIC CONDITIONS

(equipment mentioned is listed in Resources)

MYOPIA

1. Palming
2. Animal Eye Chart (no glasses)
3. Eye Dialogue
4. Brock String
5. Circle Relaxation
6. Star Relaxation
7. Ask your eye doctor for a vision fitness correction of 20/40, which can be used for vision exercises 4, 5, and 6, and can be worn for taking walks and for near focusing tasks
8. Blue-green light therapy, 15 minutes per day
9. Nutrition: Calcium, B complex, Vitamin A/Zinc, Vitamin C, Bilberry, Dr. Parcells' Thea-Lite with normalizing unit, Clorox bath for food, fasting

HYPEROPIA

1. Thumb Rotations
2. Animal Eye Chart
3. Near-far Focus
4. Brock String
5. Circle Relaxation
6. Star Relaxation
7. Ask your eye doctor for a vision fitness correction of 20/40, which can be used for vision exercises 4, 5, and 6, and can be worn for taking walks and for near focusing tasks
8. Nutrition: same as #9 above

PRESBYOPIA

1. Pinhole Glasses (15 minutes per day) for reading only
2. Brock String (5 minutes), palming (15 breaths)
3. Three-dimensional Postcards, (*see Resources*) should be done moving the card forward, backward, side to side
4. Nutrition: same as #9 above

CATARACTS

1. Eye Massage
2. Animal Eye Chart
3. Blue-green Light Therapy (20 minutes, twice a day)
4. *Succus Cineraria Maritima* (with doctor's prescription)
5. Nutrition: Food fast, Dr. Parcells' system, Bilberry, Ginkgold

MACULAR DEGENERATION

1. Eye Massage
2. Palming, Brock String
3. Circle Relaxation
4. Blue-green Light Therapy (20 minutes, twice a day)
5. Nutrition: Vitamin A/Zinc, B complex, C, Bilberry, Ginkgold, Dr. Parcells' system

GLAUCOMA

1. Eye Massage
2. Animal Eye Chart
3. Blue-green Light Therapy (30 minutes, twice a day)
4. Nutrition: Vitamin C, Bilberry, Ginkgold, Dr. Parcells' system

NOTES

1   Rowena Pattee Kryder. *The Emerald River of Compassion.* Santa Fe: Bear and Co., 1994, p.407.
2   Aldous Huxley. *The Art of Seeing.* New York: HarperCollins, 1975, p.5.
3   Janie Gustafson in *Touchstones: A Book of Daily Meditations for Men.* Center City, MN: Hazelden Foundation, 1986, Aug. 9.
4   Peter Kater and R. Carlos Nakai. *Migration* (sound recording). Boulder, CO: Silver Wave Records, 1992.
5   Frederick Franck. *The Zen of Seeing.* New York: Random House, 1973, p.3.
6   Deepak Chopra. Lecture in Albuquerque, NM, Feb. 6, 1993.
7   Lynn Andrews. "Mirroring the Life Force" in *Healers on Healing,* eds. Richard Carlson and Benjamin Shield. New York: St. Martin's Press, 1989, p.43.
8   Dr. Gerald J. Jud at Shalom Mountain Workshop, Livingston Manor, NY, Dec. 1990.
9   Antoine de Saint-Exupery. *The Little Prince.* New York: Harcourt, Brace, and Company, 1943, p.70.
10 Franck. p.96.
11 Elliot B. Forrest. *Stress and Vision.* Santa Ana, CA: Optometric Extension Program, 1988.
12 Franck. p.6.
13 Reshad Feild. *Here to Heal.* Shaftesbury, Dorset, England: Element Books Ltd, 1986, pp.109-112.
14 Franck. p.29.

15 William Padula. *A Behavioral Vision Approach for Persons with Physical Disabilities*. Santa Ana, CA: Optometric Extension Program, 1988.

16 Samuel A. Berne. "Visual Therapy for the Traumatic Brain Injured" in the *Journal of Optometric Vision Development*. Dec. 1990, pp.13-16.

17 Franck. p.130.

18 Hazel Dawkins, Ellis Edelman and Constantine Forkiotis. *Suddenly Successful*. Santa Ana, CA: Optometric Extension Program, 1991, pp.11-14.

19 Dawkins, et al. p.117.

20 Dawkins, et al. p.122.

21 *Oxford Annotated Bible*. New York: Oxford University Press, 1962.

22 John Ott. *Health and Light*. New York: Simon and Schuster, 1976.

23 Zane Kime. *Sunlight*. Penryn, CA: World Health Publications, 1980.

24 Edwin Babbitt. *The Principles of Light and Color*. Secaucus, NJ: The Citadel Press, 1980.

25 Jacob Liberman. *Light, Medicine of the Future*. Santa Fe, NM: Bear and Co., 1991, p.72.

26 Liberman. pp.75-76.

27 Franck. p.8.

28 Joseph Campbell. *The Power of Myth*. New York: Doubleday, 1988, p.88.

29 Richard Kavenar. *Your Child's Vision*. New York: Simon and Schuster, 1985, p.149.

30 Amadea Morningstar. *The Ayurveda Cookbook*. Wilmont, WI: Lotus Press, 1991.

31 Kavenar. p.156.

32 Kavenar. p.158.

33 Sharon Doubiago. "The Art of Seeing With One's Own Eyes" in *The Pushcart Prize*, X, ed. Bill Henderson. New York: Penguin Books, 1986, p.105.

GLOSSARY

Acuity: sharpness, distinctness, clearness that is dependent on retinal focus.

Age-related macular degeneration (ARMD): a vision loss in the central part of the retina.

Aikido: "the way of harmony and love" developed in this century by a Japanese master of martial arts. Aikido develops true peace within through the protection of both the attacker and defender. Energy moves in a circular flow—the attacker is welcomed, enveloped, absorbed, and then redirected by the mind and actions of the Aikidoist.

Amblyopia: also known as "lazy eye", which occurs when visual acuity is below the normal level.

Astigmatism: an unequal blur in the visual field.

Attention deficit disorder: label describing a child who has difficulty with focus and concentration.

Autonomic nervous system: part of the nervous system that governs involuntary body action such as the heartbeat, intestines, and glands. It is comprised of both the sympathetic and parasympathetic nervous systems.

Ayurveda: practiced in India for 5000 years, Ayurvedic medicine (meaning the "science of life") is a comprehensive system of medicine for body, mind, and spirit that combines natural therapies with a highly personal approach to the treatment of disease, striving to restore the innate harmony of the individual.

Binocular vision: vision that describes the eyes working together. The more the eyes work together, the better the depth perception.

Cataracts: cloudiness in the lens of the eye.

Chakra: an energy center in the body.

Chlorophyll: a plant molecule capable of absorbing light and converting it to energy for oxygen production and carbon monoxide consumption; chlorophyll is the essence of the life-supporting nutritional pattern of Earth. Especially helpful in dealing with free radicals.

Clorox treatment: a food-cleansing formula used by Dr. Hazel Parcells to remove the effects of radiation on the food as well as eliminating pesticides, germs, fungi, and metallics. Dr. Parcells recommends using 1/2 teaspoon of Clorox to each gallon of water. Timing chart follows:

heavy skinned fruits–15-30 min.   leafy vegetables–10-15 min.

thin-skinned berries–10-15 min.   root vegetables–15-30 min.

meats per pound (thawed)– 5-10 min.   eggs– 20-30 min.

Soak all food in plain water for 15 minutes after Clorox treatment.

Cobalt 60: an additive being used to extend the shelf life of food. However, according to Dr. Parcells, it kills everything it comes in contact with including living tissues.

Collagen: the connective tissue between cells

Compensating lenses: lenses that correct for blur only. They "freeze" the vision system in one place and are based solely on the visual acuity measurement of 20/20.

Convergence: eyes aim slightly inward.

Cortical blindness: the brain is unable to interpret the messages sent by the eyes.

Developmental lenses: glasses that are prescribed by Behavioral Optometrists to support and nurture an immature vision system (also called learning lenses).

Diopter: unit of measure that describes the power of a lens or optical system (such as the eye).

Dyslexia: lack of coordination and communication between body systems, often causing difficulty in learning to spell and read.

Electromagnetic energy: waves of electricity and magnetism given off by most objects.

Epithelial: protective outer layer of the cornea and other surfaces of the body.

Esotropia: an eye that turns in.

Exotropia: an eye that turns out.

Figure-ground: visual perceptual ability to see both the details and the whole picture.

Focus-in: to aim the eyes at reading distance (approximately 14 inches from the face).

Fovea centralis: the central part of the fovea which is completely made up of cone cells.

Full spectrum light: artificial lighting that simulates sunlight.

Gifted children: commonly labeled as "handicapped" or "challenged," these children with multiple handicaps or visual impairments are truly gifted and frequently very spiritually evolved.

Glaucoma: increased pressure inside the eye.

Holistic: pertaining to the whole; giving consideration to all factors including physical, emotional, mental, spiritual, social, and economic; as in holistic medicine.

Hyperopia: (farsightedness) a strain or effort in focusing.

Hypothalamus: a gland that is part of the brain that regulates metabolic processes of the body.

I.U.: International Units of measurement of food elements.

Intuition: the art of knowing without rational process.

Keratoconus: thinning and stretching of central corneal tissue which shows as a protrusion.

Kinesthetic: sensing the body through feeling; stimulated by body movements and tensions.

Learning disability: label describing a person's learning style that does not match the way he or she is being taught.

Light therapy: treatment using color to rebalance the environment within the organism.

Macula: central part of the retina where detail and clarity of sight and color awareness occur.

Macular degeneration: deterioration at the center of the retina where detail and color vision exist.

Melatonin: a hormone produced by the pineal organ that helps signal the body that it is time for sleep.

mg: milligrams

Mirroring: reporting back in an objective manner what another person has said or done.

Multi-handicapped: more than one of the sensory systems impaired.

Myopia: difficulty seeing distant objects clearly; the focus is frozen at a close distance.

Nanometer: unit of measure—one billionth of a meter.

Orthomolecular medicine: using balanced nutrition and megavitamin doses to treat mental and physical problems.

Perception: an intuition, knowledge or insight gained by perceiving. Perception is the product of perceiving. It is an interpretation of inputs which can be influenced by the accuracy or inaccuracy of inputs (from the eyes), past experiences, personality, memory, and decision-making ability. Perception is a skill we acquire and can be distorted by the mind. These distortions create warps in perception.

Peripheral vision: vision to the sides of the head (above, below, far, near, left, right, in front, and behind). Assists in balance and movement in space.

Pineal gland: the pea-size organ tucked beneath the brain, slightly above and behind the pituitary gland, that helps regulate the internal rhythm of the body.

Prana: life-force energy (Sanskrit term).

Presbyopia: blurred near objects (condition can begin around age 40).

Psychospiritual: a combination of mind/body/spirit.

Pterygium: degenerative process caused by irritation from wind or dust.

Pursuits: eye movements that are smooth in nature.

Rainbow method: a method developed by Dr. Jacob Liberman that treats a person with light therapy using all the colors of the visible spectrum and encourages full receptivity to every color.

Refraction: a specific routine of procedures that determines the compensating lens prescription of the eye.

Retinitis pigmentosa: degenerative condition where the peripheral vision begins to decrease.

Retinoscopy: procedure that measures the bending of light into a person's eyes.

Saccadics: eye movements that jump from one fixation point to another.

Strabismus: an eye turning in/out/up/down.

Suppression: an adaptation in which all or part of the visual input of one eye is prevented from contributing to binocular (two-eyed) vision.

Sympathetic nervous system: a part of the autonomic nervous system. Its main function is to prepare the body for action in emergency situations—the fight or flight response.

T'ai Chi: a centuries-old Chinese form of exercise and self-defense, T'ai Chi is meditation in motion designed to prevent illness of body and mind, and to reach self-realization. Taught as a series of "forms", the movements require relaxation, concentration, and a constant balancing of body weight.

Traumatic brain injury: trauma from a blow to the head.

Ultraviolet (UV): radiation electromagnetic waves just beyond the violet vibration of the visible spectrum.

Vestibular: concerning the aspect of the inner ear that affects balance and equilibrium of the brain and body.

Visible spectrum: electromagnetic waves seen by the human eye.

Vision Enhancement: Dr. Albert Shankman's philosophy, which states that vision takes place in the mind. It is the product of how one's mind perceives time, space, and causation. These perceptions are based on habits. Vision Enhancement is a series of vision exercises which help the person develop accurate perceptions about time, space, and causation.

Vision therapy: an organized program of activities designed to reprogram and retrain integration between the eyes, the brain, and the body. It involves working with vision on the physical, emotional, mental, and spiritual levels.

Vision: the act of sensing with the eyes, the mind, and the body. It is a learned skill that develops in a sequence of predictable stages. Sight (visual acuity, i.e. 20/20) is *one* aspect of vision.

Visual habits: these describe our visual skills such as eye movements, focusing, visual coordination, hand-eye coordination, visual memory, visual discrimination, figure-ground, form perception, and spatial relationships.

Visual learner: a person who learns best by being shown, as opposed to being told.

Vitreous: the gel-like structure found in the part of the eye just in front of the retina.

Yoga: (from the Sanskrit meaning union) a Hindu discipline of physical postures, breathing exercises and meditation practices to promote integration of body, mind, and spirit, and to enhance health and well-being.

RESOURCES

Bilberry Extract: Nature's Way Products, Inc., 10 Mountain
Springs Parkway, Springville, UT 84663, (800)866-4404

Colored Gels: Local Theatrical Supply Store
I like the CMC Color Filters colors:

Red M-112	Green M-124
Orange M-105	Blue M-174
Yellow M-101	Purple M-181

Eye Patches: Bernell Corporation, 750 Lincoln Way E.,
South Bend, IN 46634, (800)348-2225

Full Spectrum Light Products: Environmental Lighting
Concepts, 3923 Coconut Palm, Tampa, FL 33619,
(800)842-8848

Migration: (Sound recording mentioned in Introduction)
Peter Kater and R. Carlos Nakai, Silver Wave Records,
P.O. Box 7943, Boulder, CO 80306, (303)443-5617

Dr. Hazel Parcells: Parcells System For Scientific Living, 1605
Coal Street, S.E., Albuquerque, NM 87106, (505)247-2744

Parquetry Blocks and Cards: Educational Teaching Aids, 620
Lakeview Parkway, Vernon Hills, IL 60061, (800)445-5985

Physioball: Therapy Skill Builders, P.O. Box 42050, Tucson,
AZ 85733, (602)323-7500

Pinhole Glasses: Diana Deimel, 563 Third Street, Fillmore, CA
93015, (805)524-2620

Schwabe's Ginkgold: Nature's Way Products, Inc., 10
Mountain Springs Parkway, Springville, UT 84663,
(800)866-4404

Seven Pieces: Discovery Toys, Inc., 2530 Arnold Drive, Martinez, CA 94553, (800)426-4777

Spirulina: Light Force, Inc., 1115 Thompson Avenue, #5, Santa Cruz, CA 95062, (408)462-5000

Succus Cineria: Walker Pharmacal Company, P.O. Box 8080, St. Louis, MO 63108, (314)533-9600

Three-D Postcards: N.E. Thing Enterprises, 19A Crosby Drive, Bedford, MA 01730, (617)275-6960

Trampoline (Rebounder): World Wide Joy-Way Corporation, Box 39, St. Albert, Alberta, Canada T8N 2G1

Vita Drops: D.S.D. International, Ltd., 640 E. Purdue, Suite 106, Phoenix, AZ 85020, (800)232-3183

Weighted Vest: Therapy Skill Builders, P.O. Box 42050, Tucson, AZ 85733, (602)323-7500

Yoga Journal. Berkeley, CA

If you would like to find a Behavioral Optometrist in your area call or write the following organizations:

C.O.V.D. (College of Optometrists in Vision Development), P.O. Box 285, Chula Vista, CA 91912-0285, (619)425-6191

O.E.P. (Optometric Extension Program), 2912 S. Daimler Street, Santa Ana, CA 92705, (714)250-8070

P.A.V.E. (Parents Active for Vision Education), 9620 Chesapeake Drive, Suite 105, San Diego, CA 92123, (619)467-9620

College of Syntonic Optometry, Solomon K. Slobbins O.D., 1200 Robeson Street, Fall River, MA 02720, (508)673-1251

A.O.A (American Optometric Association), 243 N. Lindbergh Boulevard, St. Louis, MO 63141, (314)991-4100

SUGGESTED
READING

Andrews, Lynn. "Mirroring the Life Force" in *Healers on Healing*, eds. Richard Carlson and Benjamin Shield. New York: St. Martin's Press, 1989.

Babbitt, Edwin S. *The Principles of Light and Color*. Secaucus, NJ: The Citadel Press, 1980.

Balach, James and Phyllis. *Prescription for Nutritional Healing: A Practical A-Z Reference to Drug Free Remedies Using Vitamins, Minerals, Herbs, and Food Supplements*. Garden City Park, NY: Avery Publishing, 1990.

Bates, W.H. *Better Eyesight Without Glasses*. New York: Holt, Rinehart, and Winston, 1971.

Berne, Samuel A. "Visual Therapy for the Traumatic Brain-Injured" in the *Journal of Optometric Vision Development*, Vol. 21, no. 4, December 1990.

Campbell, Joseph. *The Power of Myth*. New York: Doubleday, 1988.

Chopra, Deepak, *Perfect Health: The Complete Mind/Body Guide*. New York: Harmony Books, 1990.

Collis, John Stewart. *The World of Light*. New York: Horizon Press, 1960.

Cousens, Gabriel. *Spiritual Nutrition and the Rainbow Diet*. Boulder, CO: Cassandra Press, 1986.

Dawkins, Hazel, Ellis Edelman, and Constantine Forkiotis. *Suddenly Successful*. Santa Ana, CA: Optometric Extension Program, 1991.

Doubiago, Sharon. *The Pushcart Prize*, X. ed. Bill Henderson. New York: Penguin Books, 1986.

Feild, Reshad. *Here To Heal.* Shaftesbury, Dorset, England: Element Books Ltd, 1986.

Feild, Reshad. *The Last Barrier.* Shaftesbury, Dorset, England: Element Books Ltd, 1993.

Forrest, Elliot B. *Stress and Vision.* Santa Ana, CA: Optometric Extension Program, 1988.

Franck, Frederick. *The Zen of Seeing.* New York: Random House, 1973.

Frawley, David. *Ayurvedic Healing.* Salt Lake City, UT: Morson Publishers, 1990.

Gawain, Shakti. *Living in the Light.* Mill Valley, CA: Whatever Publishing, 1986.

Gerber, Richard. *Vibrational Medicine.* Santa Fe, NM: Bear and Co., 1988.

Gimbel, Theo. *Healing Through Color.* Essex, England: The C.W. Daniel Company Ltd., 1980.

Goldstein, Joseph and Jack Kornfield. *Seeking the Heart of Wisdom, A Path of Insight Meditation.* Boston: Shambala, 1987.

Haas, Elson. *Staying Healthy With Nutrition.* Berkeley, CA: Celestial Arts Publishing, 1992.

Nhat Hanh, Thich. *The Miracle of Mindfulness.* Boston: Beacon Press, 1987.

Hoff, Benjamin. *The Tao of Pooh.* New York: Penguin Books, 1983.

Huxley, Aldous. *The Art of Seeing.* New York: HarperCollins, 1975.

Isaacson, Cheryl. *Yoga Step by Step.* London: Thorson Publishers, 1990.

Iyengar, B. *Light on Yoga.* New York: Schocken Books, 1987.

Jeffers, Susan. *Feel the Fear and Do it Anyway.* New York: Ballantine Books, 1987.

Jud, Gerald J. and Elisabeth. *Training in the Art of Loving.* Philadelphia: Pilgrim Press, 1972.

Kaplan, Robert-Michael. *Seeing Without Glasses.* Hillsboro, OR: Beyond Words Publishing, Inc., 1994.

Kaplan, Robert-Michael. *The Power Behind Your Eyes.* Rochester, VT: Inner Traditions, Inc., 1995.

Kavenar, Richard. *Your Child's Vision.* New York: Simon and Schuster, 1985.

Kime, Zane R. *Sunlight.* Penryn, CA: World Health Publications, 1980.

Kryder, Rowena Pattee. *The Emerald River of Compassion.* Santa Fe, NM: Bear and Co., 1994.

Lad, Vasant. *Ayurveda: The Science of Self-Healing*. Wilmont, WI: Lotus Light Press, 1984.

Levine, Stephen. *A Gradual Awakening*. New York: Doubleday Books, 1989.

Liberman, Jacob. *Light, Medicine of the Future*. Santa Fe, NM: Bear and Co., 1991.

Liberman, Jacob. *Take Off Your Glasses and See: How to Heal Your Eyesight and Expand Your Insight*. New York: Crown Publishers, 1995.

MacDonald, Lawrence. *The Collected Works of Lawrence W. MacDonald*, Vol. 2, eds. Ira Schwartz and Abraham Shapiro. Santa Ana, CA: Optometric Extension Program, 1993.

Marrone, Marcie A. "Peripheral Awareness", *Journal of Behavioral Optometry*, Vol. 2, 1991.

Messing, Bob. *The Tao of Management*. New York: Bantam Books, 1992.

Michaels, David, D. *Visual Optics and Refraction—A Clinical Approach*. St. Louis, MO: The C.V. Mosby Company, 1980.

Moore, Michael. *Los Remedios: Traditional Herbal Remedies of the Southwest*. Santa Fe, NM: Red Crane Books, 1992.

Morningstar, Amadea. *The Ayurveda Cookbook*. Wilmont, WI: Lotus Press, 1991.

Moses, Robert A. *Adler's Physiology of the Eye*. St. Louis, MO: The C.V. Mosby Company, 1981.

Mulley, Felicia Thiebeault. "Let There Be Light", *The Penn State Magazine*. March-April 1994, pp. 34-39.

O'Conner, Greg. *The Aikido Student Handbook*. Berkeley, CA: Frog Limited, 1993.

Ott, John N. *Health and Light*. New York: Simon and Schuster, 1976.

Padula, William V. *A Behavioral Vision Approach for Persons with Physical Disabilities*. Santa Ana, CA: Optometric Extension Program, 1988.

Pierrakos, Eva. *The Pathwork of Self Transformation*. New York: Bantam Books, 1990.

Schapero, Cline, Hofstetter. *Dictionary of Visual Science*. Radnor, PA: Chilton Book Co., 1968.

Selye, Hans. *The Stress of Life*. New York: McGraw Hill Book Company, Inc., 1956.

Touchstones: A Book of Daily Meditations for Men. Center City, MN: Hazelden Foundation, 1986.

Vishnudeva, Swami. *The Complete Illustrated Book of Yoga.* New York: Harmony Books, 1980.

Weiner, Michael. *Earth Medicine—Earth Foods: Plant Remedies, Drugs, and Natural Foods of the North American Indians.* New York: Collier Books, 1972.

Williams, Roger. *The Wonderful World Within You: Your Inner Nutritional Environment.* Bio-Comns. Press, 1987.

INDEX

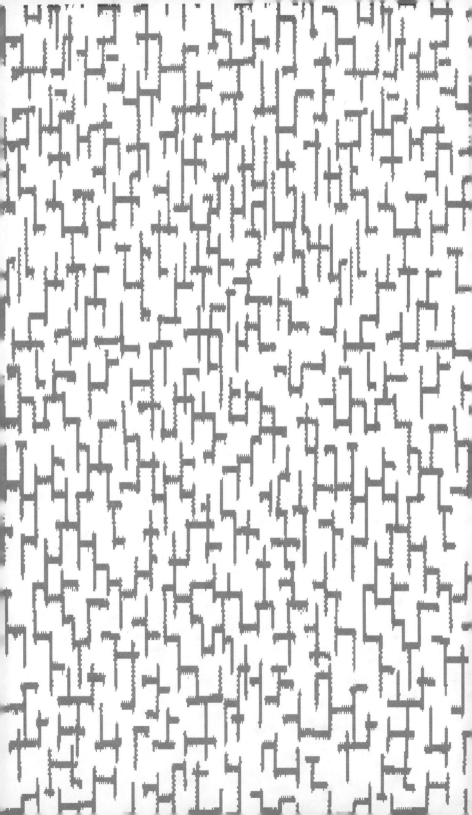